It's Just Phat, Baby

It's Just Phat, Baby

DOMINIQUE TONEY &
RIA GIBSON

It's Just Phat, Baby
Published by JM Publishing, LLC
Cleveland, Ohio, U.S.A.

www.itsjustphatbaby.com

Library of Congress Control Number 2024901440

ISBN: 979-8-9893196-0-2 (paperback)

TONEY, DOMINIQUE, and GIBSON, RIA, Authors
IT'S JUST PHAT, BABY
DOMINIQUE TONEY and RIA GIBSON

This book is printed in the United States of America.

Book Design by JM Publishing LLC

Dominique's Dedication

To my sister, Dawnnay L. Butler, I dedicate this book to your memory. You were more than a big personality, but a force to be reckoned with. Your enormous heart, dedication to faith, and willingness to assist anyone in need are why I and so many will cherish your memory.

I watched how your battle with obesity steered every decision you made from the age of five. You pushed through the pain and excelled in other areas of your life. My sister, you chose to live fearlessly despite the preconceived limitations people placed on you due to your weight. You are my shero! You taught me to "Dream Big," trust God, live life to the fullest, and look my best while doing it!

Ria and I aspire to help pre-teens, teens and young adults who have struggled with their weight and self-confidence from an early age. With you forever in our hearts, we will strive to change the way the world views and treats those who identify as or have been called "overweight." I thank you for always supporting me, and with you in mind, we hope to leave our footprints and affect change.

Affectionately, your baby sister,
Dominique

Ria's Dedication

Look, Ma, me and Nique did it! To my family and inner circle, I appreciate you all loving me no matter what shape and size I've transformed into over the years. It has been the most draining road ever! I'm ready to use the love you've given me to inspire others.

To my father, a true Leo who has always showered me with praise and healthy affection. As a dad, you have accomplished your mission with me, so don't ever think you didn't do enough. I've taken away more life lessons from you and mom than you two will ever know. My favorite quote of yours growing up was, "Don't take no wooden nickels." In other words, don't take anyone's bull***t. Become independent so you don't have to rely on anybody.

TJ, my brother, my best friend, my sounding board—sometimes the truth I do not like to hear, but most importantly, I know you want what's best for me. I also want the same for you. You've helped me navigate through all my muddy 'men' waters in life and listened to my broken records. But still, you are there, and that's something I cherish.

To the old loves in my life who didn't love me the way I deserved, thank you. You've inspired me to become transparent with my heart and reevaluate who I am as a woman. My flaws, tears, and self-questioning have brought me to this moment. This book is dedicated to reflection and growth in life and love. Hoping you all learn how to navigate through your own past trauma and learn how to love yourselves before attempting to truly love someone else.

Most importantly, to anyone who is battling obesity and issues with self-esteem, this book is for you, especially our girls and women. Do not allow anyone to subtract from your worth. God has placed you here for a purpose, young queen and young king. Keep going. Whatever you do, do not give up on—you.

Love Always,
Ria G.

Epigraph

Our book is an all-inclusive "welcoming" to those intrigued by two plus-size women finding their way through a society that defines "acceptable" body types. As women, our DNA is meticulously intended to nurture and protect, agree? As black women, the pressure to nurture, protect, raise children alone or with a mate, provide for families, become educated, battle corporate America or launch a successful business, and plan for everyone's future has exhausted our ability to protect and properly care for ourselves.

Who's looking out for us? We carry the burden of the world on our shoulders in addition to finding our place in a society handing out rules on what's in or out: phat asses, big boobs, tiny waist, perfect edges, lashes for days, perfect teeth, and a flawless coiffed style. Not to mention having the perfect career, hustle, significant other, kids, home, and car, and sometimes it is all for social media platforms. At times we neglect our inner self-care to keep up appearances for the approval of others. Hell, some of us portray images as if we have ourselves together and life is perfect when it is quite the opposite. We can pretend all we want, but we cannot run from the truth forever.

In reading this book we hope to help you navigate the trial-and-error phases of life and love. It was important for us to give people the "big girl" perspective and how the challenge of weight can impact someone's life. The experiences we have as individuals mold who we are and how we respond to situations. These moments do not define you; they are a part of your story.

Welcome to our stories.

"One of the greatest regrets in life is being what others would want you to be, rather than being yourself."
—Shannon L. Adler

Contents

Chapter 1

The Foundation

Dominique

My parents came from humble beginnings and worked hard to change their reality. Both were raised in poverty in the inner-city of Cleveland, Ohio. My mother, originally from Fayetteville, Tennessee, migrated to Cleveland at the age of five, with her parents and eight siblings. My father was born in Cleveland, Ohio and raised in a single-parent household, being one of thirteen children. Both of my parents stated they did not know they were poor or disadvantaged until they experienced the death of their mothers, as teenagers. They were stripped of their childhood and innocence, faced with the responsibility of helping to care for their younger siblings, and forced to navigate through this world with very little direction. My parents knew receiving an education was their ticket out of the poverty they experienced. After completing high school, my mother graduated from Wilmington College in two years, with a bachelor's degree in education. Shortly, after serving two years in the United States Army, my father enrolled in Cleveland State University and received a bachelor's degree in criminal justice, where he later went on to receive his juris doctorate at Cleveland Marshall Law School of Cleveland State University.

Our parents taught my sister and I the importance of having faith in God and receiving an education. Both were slim in their youth and packed on the weight as they got older. However, I cannot remember when either of them were at their smallest during my lifetime. I feared people often viewed us as the "fat" family. You know the type of family where everyone is overweight. That was my family! My mother was slightly plus, while the rest of us were obese. My father has a beer belly and is in the big and tall category. My mom was a real Halle Berry type during her young adult years. After childbirth and a love for fancy donuts, she wore and maintained a size twelve to fourteen. Both of my parents have poor eating habits. My father loves chips, pork rinds, and anything salty. My mother, on the other hand, is a very picky eater. We often joke about her poor eating habits and being a closet eater. My sister and I joined my father in his love of snacks. I believe my mother's childhood prevented her from setting boundaries and saying no to us when we wanted to overindulge on food.

Their firstborn, my beautiful sister, Dawnnay, struggled with her weight from the age of four. She never completely conquered her battle of the bulge. Dawnnay's figure was what I like to call more of an apple shape. She carried most of her weight in her upper body, mostly her back, arms, and stomach. My mother took interest in making her feel comfortable in her skin and traveled miles to the nearest plus-size stores for Dawnnay to find clothes. I remember my sister being less than enthused by the lack of color and variety in the plus-size clothing. She loved The Avenue and Lane Bryant. Dawnnay had both a creative and meticulous style. Although overweight, she maintained her hair with the latest styles and was a gifted leader and dancer. She loved red juice and Church's Chicken. We were six years apart and never missed a day of the normal sibling rivalry. She always told me she had asked our parents for me, and so I owed her for my life!

Growing up, I just knew I would be naturally pretty like my mother because during my formative years, it looked like the fat gene had skipped me. At times I was a bossy, spoiled, and mean child with the highest self-esteem. I thought I was the cutest little thing walking because I was skinny. I took pride in wearing my green and white polka dot bikini at the swimming pool. This is the first and only time I can remember having a flat stomach and feeling confident enough to wear a swimming suit in public. My ego was inflated by the compliments from family members on my small frame. Through their admiration, I learned skinny was good and acceptable. I loved to call my sister fat when we argued. It was my first line of defense. Little did I know how quickly things would change for me.

The summer before I entered third grade, boy, I gained some weight. I was no longer skinny or chubby—I was just plain ol' fat! My high self-esteem diminished with each pound I gained. My face was round, my stomach began to poke out, and my thighs rubbed together. It was as if the weight began to pack on overnight, and I no longer thought I was great. I no longer thought I was "special," and this is where my struggle with weight began. The compliments from friends and family members stopped.

I continued to struggle with my weight throughout middle and high school. In my youth, I did not have the words to express the emotional turmoil happening inside of me. Feelings of rejection, shame, confusion, and anger began to increase as I entered adolescence. I understood I was unhappy, but I lacked the insight and tools to change my situation and was too prideful and embarrassed to ask for help. Often, I daydreamed of wearing the clothes my friends wore and sharing in their confidence.

At age nineteen, I decided I wanted to fall in love with myself, determined to be comfortable in my skin. As a child, I loved riding my bike and felt this would be enjoyable and painless. I would ride the bike for an hour and find myself drenched in sweat. After completing my cardio, I would place a five to ten-pound rounded weight on my chest while I did fifty or more sit-ups. At the time I did not know what I was actually doing, or anything about building my core. But I knew I was desperate to see a different picture of myself in the mirror. I was tired of being short and stubby and felt I was too short to be plump! With consistency, the weight began to drop faster than I expected. I remember calling home and telling my parents that I lost ten pounds, with such enthusiasm. They were proud of me and rooted me on, encouraging me to continue. My sister, motivated by my determination, decided to join me. She became another cheerleader and accountability partner. I looked forward to sharing each pound I lost with her. She understood my battle with childhood obesity better than anyone. I noticed how our bond grew stronger as we focused on weight loss together. After three months of diligently working out, we lost a total of eighty pounds together. I lost thirty pounds, and my sister lost fifty. We were elated! For the first time, we felt we could conquer obesity once and for all. I remember us having a new strut that summer. Our parents bought into our healthy living, eating, and workout regime. We were excited to shop and embrace the new version of us! I learned that you can manifest the image you dream about with consistency, hard work, and accountability.

I stopped saying, "I will eat better tomorrow," making excuses and settling for being unhappy in my skin. I chose me! I chose to quiet the negative voices of defeat in my head. Over the summer I continued to lose more weight, and people noticed. They looked at me in awe and commented on how small I was. In particular, I will never forget the day my future husband Anthony walked into my dorm room with my cousin at the beginning of fall semester. I had on pajama pants and a sleeveless tank top. He looked at me and said, "Look at you with your arms out! You definitely feel more confident in your skin." Initially, I was speechless by how observant he was, but then I laughed. The truth is, for the first time since I was that seven-year-old girl in my bikini, I was confident and comfortable in my skin. I saw myself beyond the weight, reflection in the mirror, or number on the scale. I felt strong, driven, and accomplished. I learned I could do anything, and I mean anything I put my mind to.

My parents never ridiculed us about our weight and accepted us for who we were. Both told us how beautiful and intelligent we were. My sister and I saw our parents as resilient and strong. Looking back, I believe our resilient spirit, determination, and desire to improve our self-worth came from our upbringing and support rooted in our parents' unconditional love and acceptance.

Reflection:

I felt the pressure of being overweight. I wished I could walk into a room and not assume others were judging me. Like, why can't we all be skinny? My parents could have made better food choices or monitored our diets. Yet, I also realize genetics play a part in weight gain. Some people can truly eat what they want without ever gaining a pound. The complexity of it all. My family of origin laid the foundation for who I am as a person and my unhealthy relationship with junk food and becoming overweight. The mental picture

I had of myself as a child set the tone for a constant desire to be skinny and a negative self-image. The process of writing this book forced me to take a deeper look within and confront the younger version of Dominique. I found that I associated being happy with being skinny. I longed for a flat stomach and thighs that didn't jiggle. The truth is I didn't accept myself.

I support losing weight, but first you must accept yourself and all your flaws. Losing weight only fixes one part of the problem. You must confront the scars that led to emotional eating and poor self-esteem. I had to look in the mirror and embrace it all: my under belly, thick thighs, and arms. We all have positive attributes that make us special and beautiful. Wear clothes that accentuate the parts of your body that you love. Recite positive affirmations and tell yourself that you are beautiful and loved. Ignore negative feedback. Replace those negative thoughts with words of encouragement. Join a support group if you identify with being an overeater. Seek out a therapist to determine if your weight gain is connected to anxiety and/or depression. Our emotional well-being is directly linked to our physical health. When you decide to lose weight, please decide to work on yourself from the inside out. True transformation and peace happen within.

IT'S JUST PHAT, BABY

Journal Question:

Were you an overweight child? If yes, how did childhood obesity affect you emotionally?

_____

_____

_____

_____

_____

_____

_____

_____

_____

_____

_____

_____

_____

_____

_____

_____

_____

_____

_____

_____

_____

_____

"Those who judge will never understand, and
those who understand will never judge."
—Thoughts Wonder

Chapter 2

Who the Hell is Ria G?

Ria

I consider myself forever 21 at heart, but with life experiences I've been forced to reevaluate my life. My drives into the hospital (where I work as a nurse) began to consist of me pondering over my other life calling, designing my own fashion line for plus-size women; working for Gap or Target as one of the advertisement executives; becoming a freelance interior designer, a cosmetologist, or entertainer. I was beginning to feel trapped in my own life. It was one of those situations where I was asking myself, "How did I get here?"; "Where did I go wrong?" and "How the f***k do I get out?"

Once I'm dressed in my navy-blue Cherokee scrubs, I'm 90% professional at work with 10% facial expression. A true, moody Cancerian giving my thoughts away, leaving an open interpretation for the receiver of the message. Maybe I got into my career too early, and now I'm like, "What's next?" I pushed back against this uncertainty by creating new goals and started on a healing journey, bringing me face to face with my lifelong weight challenges. I have lived in a plus-size body majority of my life between sizes 18 to 20. But let me explain the "size 18." It varied from "Oh, okay, it's kinda loose," to "Ohhhh, bay-bay, this is getting kinda tight," to "Girl, just put this on reserve for a while." Weird, no matter how much weight I lost in my adult life, I never managed to get entirely out of my size 18s.

The struggle with weight loss goes back to the Catholic elementary school I attended in the late '80s and early '90s. Back then, the school checked our height and weight for scoliosis (a sideways curving of the spine) in groups of five kids at a time. The results might as well have been delivered via bullhorn for the school to know our business. Visiting the school nurse was dreadful! I remember thinking, *Please God, don't let me get weighed in front of the class jokesters.* I was already defending my ethnicity because I was light-skinned. "Are you mixed?" I was constantly questioned: "Who's white in y'all family?" or "You gotta be mixed because of your hair." "I'm black," I responded every time, and still people looked at me with question marks in their eyes. I was short and chubby with a round face and red, rosy cheeks. Bow-legged and pigeon-toed, I wore slightly turned-over orthopedic black and white saddle shoes to school every day. I paired them with a plaid jumper dress and a button-down blouse with a white butterfly collar. My mom always bought me knee-high socks, and one sock always managed to slide down more than the other. My hair was semi-long, wavy or curly, depending on the hairstyle and some kind of bow was intertwined at the top. The older girls wanted to play in my hair a lot. I recall them saying, "All this hair? You know what I would do with it?"

On scoliosis assessment days I thought, *Damn, now I gotta get on the scale with these people too!* Visibly heavier than your typical school-age or middle-school kid, there was no escaping my outward frame. The actual number on the scale was always top-secret information between me, my mom, and whoever weighed me at the doctor's office. This was my life from third through seventh grade. Nobody really clowned me too badly, but I was left to constantly wonder if this would be the day they would; this assessment always made me anxious. Impending doom settled in my chest when it was my turn to get on the scale, dreading if other kids were watching the numbers. These moments heightened my awareness that I was much bigger than the average child. Hell, this is the only reason I was determined to play basketball and softball every year in middle school. Going to practice was a guaranteed form of exercise, so why not?

There was a tremendous amount of guilt I carried for being fat and felt responsible for fixing it. I knew it wasn't "medically appropriate" to be sooo heavy that young. The feeling intensified in certain situations, like getting strapped into a ride at an amusement park; wearing a bathing suit around smaller kids; playing games that involved me running around against kids who were slender and faster on their feet; and definitely at birthday parties when it was time for food and cake (I always felt adults gave me more because I was a bigger kid). After scoliosis day at school, I'd head right to our basement with my stereo cassette player, blast my rap tapes of Naughty by Nature, Tupac, or Biggie Smalls and do jumping jacks, pushups, and run laps around the furnace. I would do this for a solid day or two until the guilt wore off and something else, like homework, began to bother me and steal my attention. The school nurse never size-shamed me. She offered me general health tips like, "Eat more fruits and vegetables, okay!" This was nothing I hadn't heard before. My doctor said it at every appointment that I can remember. Shocker.

Back in the late '80s and early '90s, being an overweight kid was rough for me. Always picked to be "It" for hide and seek. On Halloween Eve, I was pre-scolded by a pediatric nutritionist my mom found: "Now, I think you should stick to fruits and vegetables. No candy for you." Don't even get me started on gym class. Each Thursday I prayed, "Dear God, please don't let Ms. Ferguson make us run laps." Cold world, ain't it?

The worst of it, you mean to tell me that JC Penney's couldn't come up with a more discreet department section name than "Pretty Plus?" JC Penney had affordable, quality clothing and was accommodating to middle-class families, so this was our go-to shopping oasis for fashion. The clothes were decent, almost identical to the average size girls' clothes. Some styles, however, were off limits in Pretty Plus. We had a standard selection of solid colored or basic print t-shirts, blouses, printed or denim bottoms, and that was it. I remember going through the JC Penney catalog and circling all my outfits I wanted for summer, making sure to stick to the Pretty Plus section only. I loved fashion even then, circling almost the entire page! My mom would just shake her head and only ordered what I needed for the summer. Standard elastic band cotton solid shorts, sprinkled with some occasional print bottoms, and a few colored print denim shorts (my favorite). My mom always bought solid print shirts, never opting for the prints. She taught me horizontal stripes will always make you appear larger. So those were seldomly in my wardrobe. Even then I had an obsession with bright colors, especially tie-dye patterns. I think my confined school uniform lifestyle drove me to it. Maybe it was my hidden personality of wanting to live out loud, express my love for sunshine, bright blue skies, rainbows, and palm trees all the time. JC Penney is absolutely responsible for my need to coordinate though! My favorite Pretty Plus outfit of all time: lavender denim Bermuda shorts, lavender t-shirt, sleeveless lavender denim button-down shirt with white stars, paired with black low-top Chuck Taylors. Baby, I *knew* I was Cute As F***!

While I did and still love fashion, from a kid up until adulthood I had a hard time feeling the same way about my body. I would guess there are a fair number of kids and teens who share similar feelings about their own bodies or experiences, while poor diets and childhood obesity continue to increase. The same extends to obese adults in America, an increase in the number, especially among black women. The U.S Department of Health and Human Services Office of Minority Health reports African American women have the highest rates of obesity or being overweight in comparison to other groups in the U.S. (2018). For me, this statistic is true. I've been fighting the scale my entire life. I'm tired, and now I'm trying to figure this health and life thing out.

To expand on my "How the f***k do I get out of here" mind frame as of late, I must share the backstory with you: Our book idea was birthed during one of my Ria Rants with Dominique over the phone one hot summer evening. This is the beauty of having a Cancerian bestie; they don't judge you in the moment. My issue transpired from Tammy Rivera's swimsuit line for "plus-size" women (no shade, Tammy, I just gotta keep it real). I was going on about the selection of colors for plus-size women on her site. I mentioned to Dominique if Tammy had any input from her plus-size friends? Everyone knows a few curvy girls, right? From that topic, I went on to opening a store of my own for curvier women to thoughts of my own clothing line. Now we are here.

Learning how to love myself for who I am, becoming comfortable in my skin, facing the image in the mirror and accepting where I am that day whether it's good, bad, or feeling unpretty, has been one of the greatest adult challenges I've faced. Next to owing myself an apology for not putting myself first, I realized that you can change your path no matter where you are in life. That's right. I woke up one day and decided I am getting waaay too old to live in the background of my own life worried about what people may think or feel. I've learned it's okay to:

- tell people "No," or "No, I ain't got it."
- tell them why I deserve the position
- take an opportunity elsewhere if doors are not opening
- put people on the telephone block list who do not respect my boundaries, or if I need a mental break
- stop apologizing because I am not wrong all the time

I have taken the first step on the path toward living on my terms, taking the risk, and believing in my ability to achieve my dreams. Now I urge you to do the same.

Reflection:

My childhood left me with raw emotions from the opinions that other people held of me. I felt inadequate in my own skin early on, paying close attention to cellulite when I should have been focused on my Barbie collection. Learning how to become comfortable with who I am is an ongoing process to this day. Quiet time, self-reflecting, working out, reading positive quotes on Pinterest and Instagram while staying connected to people who share great laughs and elevate themselves in multiple ways helps. A lot has changed about me, and every day I'm forgiving the young girl I was because she fought like hell to become the woman she is today. I've learned if I don't respect myself I damn sure won't get it from others; the only person who will love me like me is me. Be kind to yourself because you can't depend on anyone else to do it. Even on my worst days I remind myself I am the one, never the two.

At some point a kid might say, "I can't wait to be a grown-up." Fast forward 20 years, and they're waking up at thirty-something asking, "Where did the time go?" and "Is this my life?" as they face endless bills, work commitments, family obligations, unfulfilling careers, and contemplate the dreams or aspirations they've locked in a mental file cabinet. True, some people are genuinely happy living their life like it's golden: perfect career, amazing family, beautiful home, great health, and financial stability. And then there are the rest of us still figuring our s**t out. This is okay too. No matter where you are in life you can change your path and do what makes you happy.

The Oxford Dictionary (2022) defines happy as a feeling or showing pleasure or contentment. If so, what does that look like, you know, "happiness?" I say happiness is embracing yourself and doing what's right for you. Before you start your healing journey, I want you to know a few things: Yes, you are beautiful no matter what the scale says. Yes, you are enough, no matter what asshole you encounter says on a first date or who breaks up with you. We hear you, we support you, and we want you to know we got love for you. Size doesn't matter. #Bigfacts.

Chapter 3

Vicarious Shame

Dominique

It was rare that my sister got out of school early enough to pick me up. She enjoyed walking to get me after school because she was the ultimate caregiver. I looked forward to her picking me up. I knew we would laugh while we talked about our school day. This day in particular, we decided to stop at the candy store before we went home. I didn't have much of a sweet tooth, so I was just there as her protégé, excited for our one-on-one bonding time.

We loved our rendition of a corner store located in a very small storefront. I remember walking down every aisle taking our sweet time. My sister was pretty indecisive and loved to examine each item carefully before making a purchase. Impatient, I wanted to get in and get out. I tugged on her jacket, begging her to leave the store, but she walked slowly, asking my opinion about each brand of candy. My sister hated chocolate and preferred hard or taffy candy, you know, the kind that gets stuck in your teeth. I remember snatching up a pack of green apple Now-and-Laters and saying, "Here, you love these. Let's go!" She rolled her eyes and said, "No, Dominique. I want to enjoy my snack." Which meant she wanted to choose. Frustrated, I walked around the store waiting for her to make a decision. I watched her gently place five packs of the apple and banana flavored Now-and-Laters on the counter. Finally, it was time to go!

As the cashier picked up the packs of candy and checked us out, my sister looked at him and said, "She loves candy. I told her she didn't need so much," and laughed. I looked at her, confused, stuck, and unable to defend myself. So I remained quiet until we left the store. My anger rose as I waited to leave. I wanted her to know I didn't appreciate being embarrassed or blamed for something I didn't do. She finished paying and grabbed my hand to walk out of the store. I ripped my hand from hers and stormed outside.

"What is wrong with you?" she demanded.

"Why would you say all that candy was for me?" I yelled, with a stern look on my face.

"Dominique, you don't get it. You're not fat and people won't judge you, okay! But, I didn't mean to hurt your feelings. I'm sorry."

Unsure of how to respond, I said, "Okay" and grabbed her hand. We walked home together silently, both lost in thought. I didn't realize that a year after this incident, I would gain weight and understand the fear of being teased or judged by others.

Looking back, I do not think she intended to transfer her emotions onto me. My sister, however, had gotten used to being ridiculed about her weight. Classmates and extended family members teased her despite our mother and aunts' efforts to protect her from the cruel comments of others. They jumped to her defense if anyone commented on her weight, telling people not to call her fat and teaching my sister to defend herself either verbally or physically if she felt disrespected. The comments on how much weight she gained, or the frequent comparison to those smaller than her, left a lasting impression on her young mind, making her embarrassed by her eating habits. Her pain taught me to strategically avoid the unwanted comments, stares, and judgment of those around me. She learned to beat people to the punch by diverting their attention to someone or something else. Now I see, this is a skill and defense mechanism hurt and insecure people rely on too often. I always saw my sister as "big," not referring to her weight but her personality and influence. Everyone sought advice from her, whether young or old. I often thought she was wise beyond her years. Dawnnay was my big sister, protector, strong and untouchable in my childlike innocence. Over the years, I found myself seeking her approval and satisfaction. If she approved, I somehow felt justified in my actions. She had thick skin and didn't show hurt or defeat easily. The moment in the candy store was eye-opening. For the first time I saw she was self-conscious like me. I learned how we let the judgment of others dictate the thoughts and feelings we had about ourselves.

As I have gotten older and reflected on this experience with my sister, I learned that people aren't paying as much attention to us as we think and are often too consumed with their lives to make judgments about our insecurities. I highly doubt the sales clerk at the candy store cared about how much candy my sister and I were purchasing. His attention was focused on making a sale and moving on to the next customer. The truth is we place judgment on ourselves. We allow our negative thoughts to manifest into feelings of anxiety and depression, creating a cycle of self-hate. To break this cycle, I think we have to watch the things we say to ourselves and those around us about our appearance. Why do we feel the need to say we're fat, or I need to lose a few pounds? The self-deprecating statements show those in our lives that we feel defeated and helpless. We all have something we do not like about ourselves. I have learned that everyone has a flaw or something they wish they could change about their physical appearance, personality, family, or socioeconomic status. Each of us has a quality that another person wishes they possessed. This experience taught me the importance of not jumping to conclusions and no longer feeling the need to make excuses for others to accept me because we all have flaws. We must choose happiness and be positive daily. I often tell my clients that happiness is a decision. No one is happy or filled with joy 365 days a year. Every person faces challenges, whether in their finances, family, employment, mental or emotional health. Our perception and ability to be resilient is the key to stability and joy.

Reflection:

Although a simple life lesson, I was greatly impacted by this story. My perception of my sister and genuine trust in people changed. For the first time I saw that we live in a world full of individuals who are afraid of being judged or discarded. I saw that even the strongest person cries and may suffer alone in private. Over the next few weeks, I began to watch my sister closely. Were there other things she blamed me for that I overlooked? I began to secretly judge her and resent her dismissal of my feelings. Now I see that her reaction had nothing to do with me. In fact, she became defensive and emotionally triggered by that incident as well. She was right, I didn't know what it was like to be called fat or constantly compared to others around me. I now see the constant battle she was fighting to quiet the internal voices of the negative experiences she encountered.

I never fully understood her plight, even after gaining weight the following year. I couldn't fully comprehend the pain many of us carry as a result of others' ignorance. I can empathize with my sister and understand she was tired of defending herself. She was tired of people snickering or making assumptions due to her weight. I get it and see the bigger picture. I understand it was easier to say the candy was mine. Not in an effort to hurt me, but a desperate desire and need to protect herself. With that in mind, I understand that although fragile, we often trick ourselves into thinking we are doomed and forced to suffer alone. All of us have a story, and most people are completely focused on their personal struggles. I began to realize we spend more time judging ourselves and projecting our feelings onto the outside world. Know that you deserve happiness, and it begins with a choice.

I look back on this story and recognize the power in "being yourself," whomever that is. With the understanding that I do not have to make excuses for what I eat or choose to buy. I cast down negative thoughts in my head and tell myself that the judgment of others does not reflect or determine who I am or how I feel about myself. Looking back, I see my sister needed someone to cheer her on and boost her confidence. She needed someone to encourage her to be comfortable in her skin. So I am here to cheer you on and stand in your corner, charging you to put down the feelings of shame and judgment. We all need someone to rally in our corner. We all have moments of weakness and need a strong support system in our time of turmoil and stress. Think of who is in your corner. Whether it is friends or family, is it someone that has your back no matter what? Yes, use the positive things they say about you to pull yourself up when you feel down, and if you can't think of anything, know that you are beautiful and perfect just the way you are!

Journal Question:

Have you ever felt judged by your weight or appearance?

_____

_____

_____

_____

_____

_____

_____

_____

_____

_____

_____

_____

_____

_____

_____

_____

_____

_____

_____

_____

_____

_____

_____

_____

_____

_____

_____

"Let's raise children who won't have to
recover from their childhoods."
-Pam Leo

Chapter 4

She'll Grow Out of It...
Big Beginnings

Ria

Summer babies are the best, hands down, no argument. Shout-out to all Geminis, Cancerians, Leos, and Virgos. As an emotional June baby, I've managed to change a few lives, particularly Dar (my ma) and Ira (my dad). Blessing my parents on an early June morning, I came into this world as an average-size baby: 18 inches, 7 pounds, 11 ounces, not too big or too small. I was a typical chubby baby, the kind where people say, "Aww, look at those cheeks," but somewhere between my toddler and preschool years, I morphed into this very round, cherubic girl. I mean arm rolls, thick thighs, and cheeks so big that my little white teeth and eyes sunk into my face.

Preschool was a blur. I can't recall much besides the evil teachers and disgusting food. The majority of the teachers were heavy-set and very heavy-handed. Not spelling my name right or tying my shoes incorrectly got me sent to the office and hit on my hands a time or two with a thick wooden ruler. I will never forget the seasonless, greasy baked chicken or the liver with onions. I got sick on mom's pebble-printed sheets one night after the infamous liver and onions, a pasty meat that's a great source of iron—but not for me. Who feeds that to a bunch of three-to-five-year-olds anyway?

My kindergarten experience at St. Catherine Elementary in Cleveland, Ohio introduced me to a different side of childhood obesity struggles: bullying. I *hated* this experience—throw the whole year away. The kids were cool in class, but once we hit recess—pure torture. A brown-skinned, husky, tall third grader named Antonio made my life hell. He always wore white shirts and gray or black pants and had an unkempt flat-top haircut. He would call me "fatty" or "fat girl" and pushed me up against the gray metal fence. I reported him to the recess monitor, but after a while the teacher became uninterested, almost as if she didn't believe me. Who would make that up? "Oh yes, Mrs. So and So, I'm desperately seeking out third graders to bully me." Bye, girl.

I pulled the "I'm sick card" right after the pledge of allegiance a lot. Honestly, I missed so much school; I'm surprised I passed. But hey, it was Kindergarten, no big deal. My dad's flexible work schedule became my saving grace, bailing me out of St. Catherine's and making the day ours. We would ride around, visit people, get treats (Ma did not like that), and make it over to Granny's house. Man, those were the days, especially in warm weather. I would ditch that plaid uniform dress, throw on some play clothes, and seize the day.

Mrs. Lambert mentioned my lack of attendance to my mother, so I completed my work at home. Luckily, my mom was the flashcard and workbook-type parent. Dar bought that stuff for fun (rolling my eyes), but it kinda was! The flashcards were classic shiny cardboard, white and green with simple text. I remember sitting in between my mom's legs on our big brown couch in our apartment off Sidney Avenue, enthusiastic about learning new words. With her hair wrapped in a bandana and her big gray glasses in place, Dar would quiz me and give me praise for correct answers. That was my first and last year at St. Catherine's off 116th. Just like my old coworkers would say at the end of the shift … Byeee!

Later, during my school-age years, my mother sought help from a pediatric nutritionist and cut back on the number of snacks she packed in my lunches. Instead of a ham and cheese sandwich with a snack-sized bag of Fritos, a pack of Fruit Gushers, and a Squeeze It, there was a lonely chicken sandwich on wheat, a bag of pretzels, and a Hi-C juice box. I'll never forget opening my pink and black Lisa Frank lunch box on a winter day in third grade and going to my teacher, Ms. Adams' desk, perplexed. On this particular day, there was a thermos full of Chef Boyardee and a Hi-C in my lunch box, and that was it. There had to be a mistake! Where are the chips? What happened to the cookies? I looked at Ms. Adams and said, "I think my mom forgot to pack some of my lunch." The teacher looked at me with sympathy and said, "No, Ria, I think she's cutting back on your lunch." DAMN! It's funny today thinking about how I went to that woman's desk in hopes of solving the greatest mystery of third grade: "Where the hell are my snacks?"

According to *The Journal of Family Medicine and Primary Care*, genetics is one of the biggest factors that cause childhood obesity, in addition to environmental and behavioral habits (2015). I believe habitual behaviors were the cause of sudden weight gain. Growing up, I learned "good" kids got rewarded with treats and sweets. I fell into that category. I was quiet and shy, but once I warmed up to you, I might sing you a song. My mom's co-workers loved it when I sang "Superwoman" by Karyn White. In the middle of their office, behind the thick glass windows separating the office staff from the patients, I would put on a show belting out the words to that song like a little woman scorned: "I'm not your superwoman, ohhhh no no no."

Though I was adorable, I was undeniably fat. My family loved me, but the kids at school reminded me of my oversized frame every day, snickering if I had trouble sliding out the side of the old school wooden desk; making BigFoot noises if I got up to walk to the garbage can during our quiet busy work sessions. I even felt all eyes on me when I fell down while running on the playground.

Back in the '80s and early '90s, everyone's response in my family was, "Don't worry, she'll grow out of it." My mom and dad were of average size during their late twenties and early thirties. Dar wore mom jeans and crop tops while my dad loved his shorts above the knee and button-up shirts worn the opposite (unbuttoned with gold chains glistening around his neck). I even thought, *Wow, when I grow up I'll be skinny like Mom and Dad one day.* For some reason, I thought being fat was just a phase I had to go through as a kid. Then, poof, one day I would change. Like I would magically wake up on my 18th birthday and be slim.

A child's mind is a sponge, absorbing and processing information and events throughout the course of time. What we undergo can live within and follow us into adulthood, affecting who we are and how we interact with others. Back in our day bullying existed, but it was referred to as "getting picked on" or parents/family would say "Who's messing with you at school?" The Center for Disease Control (CDC) defines bullying as a form of youth violence and an adverse childhood experience (ACE); it's an unwanted aggressive behavior that can cause physical, psychological, social, or educational harm (2021). You damn right I faked sick! I got tired of Antonio pinning me against that fence and calling me fat every day. Did I tell my parents about the third grader picking on me? I can't remember. I was such a timid kid because I was overweight. I may have mentioned it and not put much effort into my complaint honestly. Unfortunately, bullying was a part of my school and home life (certain kids on my street) during my elementary years. I'm sorry if you had to go through this too.

Antonio taught me how to run and hide from people. He set the tone for my bullying experiences, defining my role as the coward when facing my enemy. You might be thinking, "Damn, you were only in Kindergarten, ease up." But I think of how I could have kicked him in the balls, at least. Screamed, yelled—anything. But I did nothing, *not a damn thing*. In a perfect world, we like to think all children are taught to play nice with everyone. Still, the keyword is "perfect," and unfortunately, hurt people unknowingly hurt others. The older I get, the more I see this in my own relationships with family and friends.

Sitting back and observing is what I've done over the years. Paying close attention to friends or family constantly "falling out" (not getting along with everyone). People tend to lash out toward others when they have been or are being tormented themselves. Some people are not happy with themselves and will find a way to make you feel the same way too. It does *not* excuse their behavior; it just gives me something to think about when encountering their energy. This is why I've decided to limit my communication with some people and select who I share my personal life with. If your energy is not reciprocal or genuine, I'm good.

Reflection:

Funny how my mind operated as a child. I thought becoming a grown up would fix everything that presented itself as an issue in my childhood, like me being fat, and I learned that lesson the hard way because it did not. Yes, I got older and had the ability to make my own food choices, go to the gym, and participate in personal training sessions, but the weight followed me well into my adult life. I struggled to commit to lifestyle changes. My mind did not grasp the concept. I've always been more of a "quick fix" and "fast results" type of girl. Even when I'm shopping it is the instant gratification that I'm after! For example, I'm a sneakerhead so if Finish Line doesn't have my size no way am I ordering the shoe. I wanted it today, not next week! I also consider it as a sign from the universe telling me it was a purchase I did not need to make.

As I've matured, I'm learning that if you really want to change something in your life, like pursue a different career, train for an event, make major purchases like a home or car, or break away from a toxic relationship, there will be some rearranging required to make it happen. Priority number one is getting focused and depending on what my task is I struggle in this area. However, Sara Lindberg (2019) offered in the article, *Need Help Staying Focused Try These 10 Tips* and she's right:

1. Get rid of distractions.
2. Drink coffee in small doses (or other caffeinated beverages).
3. Practice the Pomodoro technique (set a timer for 25 minutes and do your thing. Take a 5-minute break and go again).
4. Put a lock on social media (use an app to block social media apps).
5. Fuel your body (foods that fuel your body with energy).
6. Get enough sleep (7 or more hours a night).
7. Set a SMART Goal (specific, measurable, achievable, relevant and timely).
8. Be more mindful (pay attention to your lack of attention).
9. Make a to-do list.
10. Focus on similar tasks (group similar tasks together).

Committing myself to some life processes has always been a struggle, like mailing birthday cards and gifts on time, returning items to FedEx or UPS for a refund before the 30-day mark, checking my mail every day, eating healthy longer than two weeks, or breaking things off with a significant other when the red flags were clear as day. I've been loyal to myself (to a certain extent) in my career, working for someone else, but when it comes down to what I really want–NO. I think about what it would feel like hitting the mega millions, writing up that two weeks' notice, and going into my manager's office the next day. He's a cool guy so I wouldn't be too harsh. Imagine me strolling into his office with my black and white checkered Vans, random Vans long-sleeve screen-print t-shirt, and navy scrub bottoms: "I know there's a staffing crisis, but in two weeks I'm out. It's been real and I wish y'all the best." Until then, I just keep showing up … a little early and ready for whatever.

Though self-commitment is hard, it's also rewarding when you accomplish what you've been working on. I've been on this journey for the last year, changing myself for the better, and I owe it to being selfish. Putting myself first. *The Blissful Mind* is a website/blog beautifully created by Catherine Beard, it is committed to helping people who feel overwhelmed and burned out determined to have fulfilling lives. In her March 17, 2021 blog, she wrote a piece titled, *How to Keep Commitments to Yourself.* Catherine offers readers some key points to get started on the road to self-fulfillment:

1. Getting in the right mindset—adjusting the negative thoughts into more positive ones
2. Repetition is key—basically, learning how to become self-disciplined and committed by establishing a daily routine.
3. Following one's North Node—(related to astrology) discovering what one's North and South nodes are and acknowledging those traits. For example, my North node is a Cancer (a warm and nurturing soul) represents the fulfillment and happiness I strive for in life. Apparently, the fulfillment I receive comes from expressing, sharing, and understanding emotions instead of placing judgment on them (sooo true). My South node is Capricorn (ughh) workaholic tendencies, being serious, the need to be in control, being

the fixer, and money means security, etc. Makes a lot of sense in my personal life. Money has never been my strong point: I've never been a stranger to go make my own. I am protective over it, but at the same time too generous with it, and not the best manager of it ... there, I said it.

One of many things I've learned lately is how to prioritize myself mentally, emotionally, and physically. This does not happen overnight. It is a process I work at daily, a true commitment to self. I've sought counseling for my mental well-being. Honestly, my best friends needed a break from my personal drama. It's good to get unbiased feedback from a licensed professional who could see what I was going through with a clear lens. I've rearranged my life to enhance all three areas (mental, emotional, and physical): I've had weight loss surgery; learned more about health and wellness to help myself and others (in the future); maintained a workout and nutrition regimen; relocated to my hometown for the time being; changed jobs to leave the past in the past; utilized the "blocked list" because my boundaries are important; picked up a second job for extra cash flow; worked on additional certifications and personal projects. Self-prioritization is not all serious business either, it's important to include activities that make you just feel good about yourself, like routine upkeep such as manicures or pedicures, eyebrow maintenance, a massage every one to three months, or an occasional shopping trip to Sephora for new lip wear.

With all this being said, I'm not that same little girl I was in Kindergarten (Thank God), just standing there all helpless. I've decided, "F*** that! I'm better than this. I got work to do."

IT'S JUST PHAT, BABY

Journal Question:

Think back to a time when you were bullied? Who was your aggressor? Was this emotional, mental, or physical? How did you respond? How has this affected you today?

_____

_____

_____

_____

_____

_____

_____

_____

_____

_____

_____

_____

_____

_____

_____

_____

_____

_____

_____

_____

"Bullying is not a reflection of the victim's character,
but rather a sign of the bully's lack of character."
—Unknown

Chapter 5

New School
New Attitudes

———

Ria

First Grade

I was looking forward to the new school building, new uniform, and fresh faces at CKS elementary. I remember Mom walking me to the first-grade line, holding my hand. Imagine me, bow legged with a bright red ribbon in my hair, half up half down hairstyle (ponytail to the side), a white short-sleeve butterfly collar shirt, green and navy plaid uniform dress, black and white Oxford shoes while carrying a red Garfield the Cat lunchbox.

Mom kissed me good-bye, marking the beginning of eight years of learning that would lay the foundation for my friendships, romantic relationships, and academic success. I was about ninety pounds, but in pictures I did not appear as heavy. Well, according to picture day 1989 (JCPenney purple and black sweater skirt set, black and white bow in my hair, and for some reason I was very tan like I vacationed in Hawaii all summer). Anyway, there were two girls in the class I identified with because they were chubby: Malorie and Dakita. But Dakita had the nerve to be evil! I mean, perhaps she was having a tough time at home, which proves the theory to be true: Hurt people hurt people. She tried me any chance she got. Simple things like rolling her eyes, snatching things out my hand, the audacity. Dakita, being a bigger girl herself, did not necessarily make fat jokes toward me, but she wasn't a nice girl period. Of course I never said or did much back in response, too focused on being the "good girl" in class. I never forgot about her and wondered why as a fellow big girl would she go out of her way to be so mean to me? There weren't that many chubby kids in class. We were the minority and needed to stick together, you know? Malorie was cool, though. She was like a carefree spirit. She always laughed in a way that made you feel like it was just you and her in the room; no one else mattered.

Second and Third Grade

By third grade, my weight was consistent, and I was keeping it cute in clothes from the "Pretty Plus" section of JCPenney. My mom would get frustrated sometimes in those tan-carpeted dressing rooms. Whenever we had to go up a size, it felt like she was disappointed that I was getting heavier. She sighed a certain way as she tried zipping my pants up or tugging the waistband for a fit check. Now, my immediate family loved me for me. I honestly cannot remember anyone poking fun or saying hurtful things out loud anyway. If anything, aunts and uncles would tell my mom, "Don't worry, she'll get taller. She'll grow out of it." Or they'd use the infamous line in our family, "She's just big boned. That girl is solid." Family always kept my cousins and me fed on the weekends, in the summer, and on holidays, sharing "cute" baby stories about me being fat: "We were eating breakfast one morning and the next thing I knew, I looked down and saw this little hand grabbing a sausage off my plate!" It was my plump hand. My parents and family treated me like a regular kid. I was in my own head more often than not in certain situations, worried what someone was thinking about me.

I tried hard to be active at home, riding my bike, and/or playing kickball with kids on the street. It was constantly on my mind to be a "normal size" kid. Whenever spring and summer made its way back to northeast Ohio, it reminded me of the *Rocky* movies (particularly *Rocky 2*) and how it was time to start training: "Okay, I'm going to ride my bike up and down the street ten times after school and run up and down our steps ten times before bed." I watched *Video Soul* and *Rap City*, attempting to dance the fat away in our back room when the weather got too cold. Babes, I am not new to this physical fitness game! My immediate family embraced who I was, but it was a nagging pain I felt in social gatherings where anyone's eyes could see what I was eating or monitor how much. My elementary school did not have a cafeteria, so we ate our lunch privately at our wooden desks with small random chatter.

In my neighborhood, there weren't too many birthday parties or get-togethers held inside peoples' homes. We were more of a "let's go to the corner store" or "oooh, here comes the ice cream truck" crowd. Of course I had moments where I was too shy to really eat in front of my peers. They were predominantly male, one whom I liked *a lot*. But we shared fun times over classic urban delicatessens like chico sticks and Faygo pop; nacho cheese Doritos with souse meat; Little Hug barrel fruit juices and splitting home cooked burgers on white Wonder bread.

Around this time, I developed boy crushes at school. (Call me fast, go ahead!) I even had a slender, tall boyfriend named Scottie. I may have been chubby, but ya girl was always cute. I've always paid attention to my outward appearance: Absolutely *no* body odor, dirty shoes or shoestrings, or wrinkled clothing. My hair was neatly combed (a ponytail with a bang to the side). My dad was always sharing stories from high school with me. Everyone went to school dressed "sharp," and he was one of them. His mother was very particular about her home and personal hygiene, so growing up I learned a lot from her. My grandmother, a very meticulous woman, would be donned in her classic floral housecoat and leather house shoes; she wore her hair with a curly slicked-back ponytail like Megan thee Stallion style, "feeling like I'm Ice-T." I knew people were already going to judge me for being a fat girl, a heavy girl, a chubby girl. They could never say I was funky, musty, or sloppy. If anything, I was going to be that cute big girl who was neat, matching, and clean.

Now getting back to slim Scottie and our short-lived school affair. We kept each other's yearbooks and school-embroidered marker holders in each other's desks. No one else knew. But I wondered, *Was our school-age love classified information because he was ashamed of my size?* We were young, so we were not having deep conversations. I was definitely one of the chubbier girls in class and presentable. Crisp catholic uniform dress with butterfly collar shirts creased to perfection, who could resist? Well, at the end of one school day, he dropped me … out of nowhere. He didn't say it directly, but we were cleaning out our desks, and he gave me my yearbook back and asked for his. And here is where my first dose of heartbreak settled in. Scottie and I remained friends of course, in a small class of kids under twenty it was unavoidable. It was cool. We were young and let's be honest, we were secretly housing school supplies inside each other's desk! I will not deny my second grade heart was hurt. It was unexpected and out of nowhere, so imagine the shock! However, I was resilient even then. I could do better than that! There were boys on my street who I got along with anyway, so who needs "so and so!"

The boys I grew up with became more like cousins ... well, at least two or three of them. One had my heart for years, and there was one who made my life hell. I was every bit of a "fat white girl" whenever we got into it (mostly during street games of kickball or hide and seek). His words sat with me during my younger years, adding to my insecurity about my size in comparison to everyone on the street. I asked God, "Why do I have to be sooo light skinned? I'm tired of telling everyone I'm black and all they do is second guess me." Some days I didn't even go outside if my cousin and I were at odds. That made everything worse. Darnell was mean but he was brutal, jumping on the verbal bandwagon and wanting to fight me. I will be the first to admit I was no Mike Tyson growing up. Hell, call me Scary Mary. My anxiety would shoot through the roof, gathering in front of someone's house for the infamous pick to be "It" for hide and go seek, knowing my fate for the day. I was the second chubbiest and slowest kid on the block. I was always "It" for hide and go and seek. Looking back on the situation, Darnell may have had a reason to be mad and take his anger out on me. As kids we didn't understand what our peers experienced behind closed doors. Some children struggled in school, felt inferior playing sports, shared a bed with multiple siblings, or never experienced a vacation or a fun day out (e.g., going to Chuck E. Cheese). Perhaps more often their utilities were off in the house, or were being raised by someone other than mom or dad, or lacked love and attention from family. The life my parents and other family provided me was simple: I had my own room with a full-size bed from the age of two, cable TV with occasional access to HBO or Showtime, trips to the movies and the mall, going to Red Lobster, one summer vacation a year within the United States, or going to Geauga Lake (one of Ohio's nostalgic amusement parks) once a year. Someone on the outside looking in may have thought, *She is living the life.* Either way, Darnell, I forgive you. Those comments contributed to my few years of self-doubt, constantly comparing myself to other females. Running the hamster wheel constantly in my mind: I am too fat, or why can't I be darker? Why can't I just look like everyone else slender and brown without further questions. It almost felt like a target on my back at times, depending on Darnell's mood. Thank you for helping me realize after many years, the problem was never me. It was you.

My street crush, Young Fresh, was always clean from head to toe, literally. He was the only ten year old at that time who wore Ralph Lauren Polo. His shoe game was always up-to-date Jordans, Nike Air Raiders, and the infamous Nike Penny Hardaway's that were stolen from a Cedar Point water ride. I still owe him one.

We were nine or ten years old when my parents took me, one of my girl cousins, and Young Fresh for a summer day of rides and fun at the infamous Cedar Point Amusement Park. I remember feeling soooo excited about this trip! Time alone-ish with my neighborhood sweetheart away from our usual routine of kickball and bike riding! I also can't forget feeling uneasy next to my much slender cousin. Her bathing suit was definitely cuter. There I was standing in lines to ride rollercoasters with the two of them, dreading the moment we hit the water ride. My bathing suit was hideous: Pretty Plus special (a black and navy one-piece with peach floral side panels). Ugghh! Picture me standing there, a chubby, sweaty girl with a long braided ponytail standing next to her much skinnier cousin in front of her street crush. There is nothing worse than wiping away your top lip every few minutes next to the boy you like.

Young Fresh was something even then. He had these slanted eyes that always made my heart gasp if I stared directly for too long. He was the start of my "butterflies over boys" phase. They say you never forget your first kiss: awkward, exciting, and leading this young Cancerian into her own "when we grow up thoughts." One fall evening after a bike ride, Young Fresh offered to help carry my heavy-ass mountain bike into the basement. After a brief prep talk about kissing, "it" happened (kissing sounds). He was definitely into it more than I was, but mostly because I was such a chicken! Nervous about getting caught by whoever was home that day, I wondered if I was doing it correctly.

He always made me feel special in his own way. I will never forget around the age of six or seven years old, my cousin and I walked up the street role-playing in our own world with our baby dolls in strollers. Mom managed to find me one of the last African American Baby Alive dolls for Easter. I took extra good care of her, head to toe. Well, on our stroll, Young Fresh and Ducky were outside just kinda standing there on the sidewalk. With the greatest sense of pride, Young Fresh yelled out, "Ria's baby is my baby." It was bold. He was the first male (besides my dad) who ever bought me jewelry, a tennis-style bracelet designed with maybe Xs and Os (we were about ten years old). If anyone knew my mother, hell even now, they knew she did *not* let me keep it! I remember her words like yesterday, "You are too young to be accepting gifts like this from boys." I felt bad about it for the longest time. As warm and fuzzy as he made me feel, I don't know if a part of me felt it couldn't be true. I kept asking myself, *Why does he like me sooo much?*

Even Young Fresh's haircuts were different. I will never forget his s-curl look paired with a gold hoop earring, and he managed to pull it off. I think he set the bar high for everyone on our street. If he was coming outside, I paid extra attention to my outfits. Sometimes I thought I wasn't good enough for Young Fresh. My limited hairstyles, Pretty Plus clothes, and mediocre shoe game back then said so in my mind. In reality, as we got older our interests were different, and we grew apart. But I always thought of him and "what if . . ."

In third grade I really began to thrive academically, making up for being a physical failure, I suppose. Even at a young age I thought, *If I can't be a normal-size kid, I gotta be good at something else!* So school became my focal point. It was something I could control, and I enjoyed praises for doing well. There was always some competition in my peer group. One of my classmates was extremely smart, and I prayed many a night for her mathematical wit. She always "got it," no matter what. My best friend at the time was also smart, and when I didn't feel as adequate on a test or two, there was always my other friend who made me realize imperfection is okay. Besides, it was too much pressure for third grade.

Reflection:

Our childhood foundation is vital to our adulthood. A group of medical researchers created an Adverse Childhood Experiences (ACE) score to connect and measure potentially traumatic events: violence, abuse, or growing up in families with mental illness or substance use (2022) to the health risks and behaviors in adults. Ready for this? According to the CDC, ACEs are common and over time the effects can negatively impact physical and mental health (diabetes, heart disease, poor academic achievement, and substance abuse), which makes sense. I also learned females (African Americans and Hispanics) are at greater risks for experiencing four or more ACEs (CDC, 2022). This outcome is scary if you think about it. One incident, in my opinion, can affect you to the point where you are no longer the same. A part of you may die that day, and your trauma is born.

We experience situations as children intertwined with emotions that can become a part of our adult identity. The name calling, constantly being "It" for hide and go seek, or being the easy target for jokes because I was the heavier girl are memories that followed me as an adult woman. Depending on where she was and who was around, that shy, fat girl became the overweight, anxious, and sometimes insecure woman who constantly wondered if someone was thinking, "Yeah, she's too short to be that big," or "She's cute, but would look even better if she was smaller."

I've struggled with weight in adulthood as I did in my childhood, but earning my certifications, highly satisfactory or outstanding on performance evaluations, and doing well in my career and the experiences I've had with the people I've met along the way have given me a sense of pride. Today, I enjoy the positive praise I receive for being a "good" nurse. It gives me the same feeling it did years ago in elementary school. But now my inability to fit in physically along with the shame I carried around for failing in this area has taken a backseat.

With age, it becomes clearer that the best competitor to have is yourself. End of discussion. This is healthy for the mind, body, and spirit. If you're not looking at yourself in the mirror, having honest discussions like, "Okay, what do we need to change?" Or my favorite, "Get your shit together," you're doing yourself a disservice.

I looked myself in the eyes and took ownership of all my nonsense and determined what I wanted moving forward. I learned what works for someone else may not work for me, so it took time to discover my "thing." I learned how to tap into who I am by doing things that fuel my competitive spirit, like therapy every two weeks, working out three or four times a week, creating music playlists, therapeutic shopping if extra money permits (candles from Bath and Body Works), and taking long showers.

That's what I'm on, baby—good vibes.

Accepting what has happened, what is going on in the present, and claiming the future—is that easy? Helllll *no*! That's why some of us are still where we were three years ago. But when you're ready to seek change, go for it. Block out negative vibes to make room for positivity. This means cutting folks off, leaving some bad habits behind, adopting a new mindset—and don't forget about believing in yourself.

When you are going through personal storms like bad breakups, job loss, conflicts with family or friends, or weight gain or loss, leave Facebook, Instagram, Snapchat, and Twitter alone! Trust me on this. I know from personal experience that it helps. Delete the apps for a while. Why? These social media platforms have the potential to drive a fragile mind into a deeper rabbit hole of helplessness. Feeling like your life is in shambles, unbalanced shit is happening left and right, and the reflection in the mirror is a hot mess. Being glued to your device, watching all the great aspects of someone else's life is no bueno. Consider social media a temporary zone of self-destruction.

Sometimes these platforms leave us questioning every decision we've ever made, beating ourselves up over the shareable size bag of peanut M&Ms we devoured during last night's pity party, or replaying Mary J and Jazmine Sullivan on iTunes while contemplating texting people who are not thinking twice about us. Hunnie, NO. Not today.

Journal Question:

Can you think of a time when you first experienced rejection? How did it make you feel? Did you use the experience as an opportunity to put energy into something else? Was it positive or negative?

_____

_____

_____

_____

_____

_____

_____

_____

_____

_____

_____

_____

_____

_____

_____

_____

_____

_____

_____

"If you live for people's acceptance, you
will die from their rejection."
—Lecrae

Chapter 6

First Day of School

Dominique

O n the first day of third grade, I entered the cafeteria wearing a white blouse, black skirt, and loafers, ready to accept my new title as a third grader. I smiled at familiar faces and darted off to talk with friends I had missed over the summer. When I walked down the aisle I overheard Brian, my first crush from kindergarten, talking about me to another boy. "Look at Dominique. She's fat now. She used to be pretty," he whispered. I pretended not to hear him and quickly walked back to my seat. What he said haunted me from that day forward.

Up until then I saw myself as attractive. My looks were the foundation for who I *thought* I was. Back then I thought being "pretty" determined how much you were liked and accepted by others. I assumed I was accepted by others based on the compliments I received and/or words my parents and family members used to describe me, such as: adorable, cute, and pretty. The attention I received from boys in class solidified the perception I had of myself. My self-acceptance was rooted in how I felt other people saw me.

This single event created a chain reaction in how I viewed myself. My newfound identity became rooted in shame, rejection, and fear—the fear of not being accepted by others and of not measuring up or being as desired as the other girls in class. My heart was crushed after I heard Brian's comment. I immediately thought, *I'm ugly now?* I hadn't realized how much weight I had gained until he made that remark. My parents didn't comment on my weight. They never made me feel bad about myself or suggested that I lose weight. I now see that my parents overcompensated by telling me how beautiful and special I was. They understood the challenges my sister and I faced as overweight children and attempted to boost our egos with positive affirmations to overshadow the painful comments of others. Although I felt insecure being overweight, my parent's unconditional love and acceptance kept me from falling into depression. I never questioned whether they loved or accepted me. An unconditional love I found in my relationship with my immediate family.

What Brian said diminished my once-inflated ego. I no longer saw myself as attractive and began to question how everyone saw me. *Did everyone think I was fat and unattractive?* I withdrew socially and feared speaking up for myself. Prior to this incident, I was outspoken and confident. But afterward I found myself following the crowd in an effort to belong. I became the class clown, using my wit to overshadow my insecurities. For my peers, I learned to put up a tough facade to appear funny and unbothered by the teasing I occasionally endured. I hid the quiet tears, shame, and self-doubt from those around me. At that young age I became mindful of my clothes and the way I looked, spending hours in the mirror contemplating what I could wear to appear smaller.

As an adult, I recognize that I started to associate being skinny with being pretty at the age of eight. I identified being "overweight" as being damaged goods, believing I was no longer beautiful or likable. My childlike innocence was swiped away in a moment. On that day, I began hiding behind a mask of pain, secretly seeking the acceptance of others. I should have loved myself when others passed judgment. When you have a solid foundation and are taught to believe in yourself as a young child, those words of rejection become more difficult to receive and lose their power. But, remember the old nursery rhyme, "Sticks and stones may break my bones, but words will never hurt me." How many of us have found just how untrue this saying is? The truth is words cut far deeper than any physical wound or scar. An emotional wound can last a lifetime. We allow those words of hurt and rejection to penetrate our minds, hearts, and souls, building a wall of defense that leaves us trapped in that moment. A moment defined by hurt and trauma. Trapped until we make a decision to forgive.

This was my first personal encounter with the harsh reality of being overweight. Prior to this moment, I recognized how the world viewed my sister due to her weight, but now this was my reality too. I realized that not only was I being judged for being chubby, but I was no longer viewed as attractive or socially accepted by my peers. As the anxiety increased, I remember feeling like something was stuck in my chest while I listened to Brian's comments. I felt helpless and vulnerable. Pushing back tears, I walked away and wallowed in self-pity.

You see, this story taught me that the harsh words of others can change not only the way we view ourselves but the direction of our lives. I often wonder how my life would be different if I did not experience this encounter with Brian. Would I have remained innocent and oblivious to my weight gain or the way my peers saw me? Would I have held my head high and walked with a sense of confidence instead of shame? One will never know, but one thing is for sure: his stinging words peirced me internally. This childhood encounter has followed me into my adult life. To this day I shudder at the idea of walking past a crowd. My anxiety often overtakes me with negative thoughts. Self-doubt creeps in, and I wonder if they are whispering about my weight or overall appearance. I know how foolish this may sound to someone, but this is my reality. It is true that words not only hold power but leave deep wounds and scars. I have also learned that in order to move forward, we must forgive our offender and ourselves. Today, I forgive Brian, and I choose to forgive the eight-year-old version of myself. I choose to move forward and recognize that my worth, beauty, and happiness are not determined by my relationships with others but by the relationship I have with myself.

Reflection:

Too often, we, as women, allow society to dictate how we view our bodies and overall self-worth. The lies we tell ourselves as children continue to mislead us into adulthood. I waited my entire life to grow out of my "baby fat," and guess what. I didn't. Complete opposite! I became more round in my frame. However, I did learn my unhealthy relationship with food partnered with low self-esteem grew with every pound I gained along the way. In an effort to hide my true emotions, I found solace in food. I realize I should have been honest with those around me, about my struggles with weight and self-esteem. Instead I chose to hide behind a false persona of being funny, strong, and unbothered by my weight. I wish I could tell my younger self the importance of living your truth. The importance of asking for help and letting those around you know that you are unhappy or struggling. I feared being seen as weak if I told my family and friends. Often, I thought I was drowning emotionally, struggling to belong with thoughts of inadequacy.

So while I continue to embark upon a new journey of self-love and acceptance, my advice to you is "Stop Hiding!" As people, specifically women, we must acknowledge who we are unapologetically and become healthier for ourselves. On that note, I leave you with this:

You are altogether beautiful, my love. There is no flaw in you.
Song of Solomon 4:7

This Bible verse shows me that we are all beautiful to God. When he looks at you and me, he does not see our imperfections and mistakes. He sees the treasure that he created. He sees our gifts and the promises he has in store for us. The talent each one of us has to leave our imprint on the world. This verse helps me to love myself and know that I too have purpose.

"Confront the dark parts of yourself, and work to banish them with illumination and forgiveness. Your willingness to wrestle with your demons will cause your angels to sing."
—August Wilson

Journal Question:

Can you recall a time when you were deeply hurt by someone's words? If yes, reflect on their words and why they hurt you.

_____

_____

_____

_____

_____

_____

_____

_____

_____

_____

_____

_____

_____

_____

_____

_____

_____

_____

_____

_____

_____

"A tongue has no bones, but it can break a heart."
—Unknown

Chapter 7

Puberty Strikes

Ria

etween the ages of ten to twelve years old, I learned what clothing worked best for my frame and what did NOT. Certain materials chaffed my skin. It was dreadful. Perfect example, I avoided all fabric tights for the longest time, especially cable knit, like the sweater. Other fabrics were comforting to my heavier frame, such as 100% cotton. It was lightweight and breathable and always presented the cooling factor. Nothing was more embarrassing for me than being plus size and sweating profusely on a hot day. Sweat stains on display under your butt creases or underarms while trying to look your best. I felt people associated me with a BBQ pig logo from a random restaurant.

Don't get me wrong, in all my crazy thinking, my mom was there for me during my struggles of being a fat kid who was being teased, or feeling like an outcast at times, or frustrated with fashion. But at the end of the day, my mom wasn't a "heavy kid" growing up. I was my own advocate when we shopped for my clothes as I learned what flattered my round frame and what did not. However, she offered one solid piece of advice: "Horizontal stripes will make you look bigger so avoid those." She understood and listened, thank God.

During this era, I took on certain rites of passage like hair styling and preparing my own clothes for school and developing my own style. I didn't have much to work with since I went to Catholic school, so shoes, socks, and hair scrunchies birthed my "Ria G" style. As a Pretty Plus child, I was self-conscious about hygiene and maintaining a neat appearance because it provided a sense of security and control. My dad also played a role, instilling the importance of self-presentation, especially in public. He is from an era where it was not uncommon to wear a three-piece suit in high school. He was meticulous about everything: jeans and shirts were Carhartt, shoes: Redwing, socks: Gold Toe, cologne: Grey Flannel, and he always tucked his undershirt in his underwear! Weird, but I get it. I had my father's derriere and understood why he did it. Even now when I bend over in my patient's room to empty a Foley catheter, I refuse to have the infamous "plumber's butt crack." You will see an Old Navy camisole tucked tightly into Victoria's Secret briefs on days I'm wearing my not-so-favorite Cherokee scrub pants.

My classmates were also coming into their own. Developing physically, taking more pride in their appearance, and talking more about the opposite sex. The funny thing is our classroom did not have many options. We had about six boys to fifteen girls, and we were a small group. There was a clear divide among us: the pretty girls, the rivals, the smart kids, and the kids who talked too much. You know, the ones who always had a response when the teacher gave directions and always had something to say.

Some of us started looking at the boys in sixth grade differently—including me. I'm "some of us." Despite my early struggles with body image as I grew older, I was able to see beyond people's shiny exterior and explore the connections we developed through our interactions. It was how they made me feel when we talked for hours over the cordless phone that mattered most. The moments of laughter, them opening up about their fears and shedding tears let me know they had real emotion. More importantly, it made me realize how vulnerable they were and how comfortable they felt with me. That meant more than if the shoes they had on were Jordans versus Nike Trainers.

I had the biggest crush on AC—he was my boyfriend. He was chubby, well-groomed, a comedian, an artist, and was soooo cute to me. AC's acceptance of my appearance also heightened my attraction toward him; he made it quite obvious he was "in love," smiling ear-to-ear when we saw each other, waiting for me every morning, and the exchange of phone numbers! Once we crossed into telephone territory, it was official. My mother restricted my talk time to weekends. Her goal was to keep me focused, and that was smart, Mom. Well played. Back then, I always thought my mom was an evil wizard depriving me of simple pleasures. No, she was protecting me from bullshit, and it worked. I never fell behind in my books. She placed a certain type of fear in me by keeping it real.

But back to AC … yes. AC wore these black-and-white Reebok trainers for gym class and basketball. Chile, I begged my mom for the same pair. I picked an alternative color, white, blue, and black. He was best friends with my play cousin, so these were all major wins for me. AC would wait for me in the drop off area in front of our school's church, and we would walk to the morning lineup together. That was romance, okay! My heart rate would beat above normal (full sinus tachycardia), anticipating his big shiny cheeks by the bushes or watching his big Atlanta Falcons coat up the hill.

As my feelings for AC grew, so did my attention to details and what the opposite sex might like, for example flavored lip gloss. I remember Mom randomly buying me things like Lip Smackers bubble gum gloss. One day on our walk to the line, he kissed me (nothing messy, people! We were young.), and he was impressed by the bubble gum flavor and kiss. Mental note to self: All lip gloss must be flavored for my secret AC kisses. Check.

In school, we were secret lovebirds: meeting at the water fountain just to say hi; walking by each other's classrooms taking advantage of the open doors to make each other laugh, making goofy faces; sitting by each other when our classrooms connected for movie afternoons. I mean, we didn't even need to sit directly next to each other, okay. It was enough to be in the vicinity of desks! To see his crisp baby blue oxford shirt, black tie, and big white smile with those chubby cheeks sent me over the top! My middle school heart was in love for sure. AC had dope skills with pen and paper, a real artist. For my birthday, he drew the album cover of Outkast's *Southernplayalisticadillacmuzik* flawlessly. Throughout our relationship, AC would often draw me pictures. Once in a blue moon he would find a way to sneak them into the side of my desk. Such a clever and romantic gesture, right! Our classrooms would switch room to room for different subjects making this act of love possible. The Outkast drawing was special. With pride I hung it in my room, finding space for it alongside my *Right On* and *Yo! MTV Raps* posters that littered my baby blue wall. I always thought he should draw for a textbook company or comic books.

Honestly, I can't remember what caused the premature breakup between AC and me, the details locking our puppy love chapter in the pound. But whatever happened hurt me to my core. His actions pushed me to the unthinkable in his eyes: tearing his infamous Outkast picture off my wall and ripping that bitch up into tiny pieces. He was livid, and I was relieved. The beginning of unhealthy coping mechanisms … destroy and decease.

Between sixth and seventh grade after the AC breakup, I started talking to Hunter. He was a year ahead of me, tall with hot chocolate skin, wavy black hair, and well known for his "big nose." Pimples attack us differently in our teenage years, and his were always right on his nose. He always told me I was his "Tia Carrera," which was odd because I'm not Asian, Blasian, or skinny. But with that comparison, I felt beyond confident. Hunter was also attracted to thicker girls, so it was a win for me. This is why talking with him over the phone became easy; he made me feel comfortable, and boy did we talk. We spent hours on the phone laughing while on three-way calls with his best friend and my best friend at the time. He even shed tears about his home life. I was so in awe of Hunter. After school I rode my bike to meet him at Forest Hills Park for ten minutes of kissing and after-school chit chat about how much we liked each other.

We even shared the mutual state of Virginia where our extended family members lived. His older sister lived in Virginia Beach, the same area as my favorite aunt and uncle. We were able to meet up one summer and go to the movies. I remember my little cousin tagging along. It was a little awkward, but baby, back in my day, you brought whoever along to be with your bae. I mean, don't get me wrong. AC and I always had a connection, but Hunter was his replacement at the moment. Our romance was not one I boasted about because he was considered a "cornball" or "lame" to his counterparts: he was not the best on our school's basketball's team. He didn't have the latest Nikes or Jordans, and was not a class clown, attention-seeking kid like most boys in his class. I got to know the real Hunter, and that's what got me. He was genuinely goofy, warmhearted, and did not make me feel self-conscious about anything. AC had older brothers who talked to him about the oddest things, like cellulite on women. I remember talking to him on the phone after school one day looking in the mirror during the cellulite conversation and thinking, *Damn, I have cellulite. This is bad.* I didn't experience moments like this with Hunter.

Reflection:

Middle school is one of the most challenging times in our lives. It is a time of finding our place among peers while trying to discover who we are as we transition from child to young adult. It's one of the most confusing times we experience in life. We are more in tune to adult conversations and learning about all types of responsibilities while trying to be a kid at the same time. STRESSFUL. Add the way we often scrutinize our bodies at this age to the mix, and it's easy to see why many of us carry our childhood struggles into adulthood. According to a February 2021 article entitled *Body Image (Children and Teens)* on the *familydoctor.org website*, children's opinions about their bodies form as young as three years old and can create body image issues. The way children perceive themselves can affect different aspects of their lives, creating lifelong social consequences like a reluctance to try new things in general, even seeking a higher education.

Watching videos on *Rap City* and *Yo! MTV Raps* heightened this plus-size girl's confidence in the mirror. Perfect example, I was beginning to realize my bigger butt was actually a "good thing" and nothing to be ashamed about. Back then, music entertainers were not yet creating videos with women shaped like Meg the Stallion and Lizzo. Butt enhancement procedures (e.g., the Brazilian butt lift or butt implants) were not something women boasted about having done. Images across our screens were more light-skinned or light-brown Jane Fonda types: petite frames, slim waist, and proportioned backsides to match. Having a larger derrière was slowly beginning to create a buzz for celebration. Even so, butt size in the '90s does not compare to the Dr. So & So physiques today. That is a fact, and I'm more than willing to argue.

I found my younger self dating people for who they were and how they treated me (the second part is more important than the first). Even though I was attractive, it was never enough to ignore that I was also heavy-set, chubby, plus-size—however you want to chop and screw that up. Some boys were going for average size or slimmer girls. I got in where I fit in. I liked the boys for who they were, and I expected the same.

This period in my life was the beginning to an ongoing journey of connecting with my bad-ass inner confidence. Discovering the "shero" who lays dormant underneath the insecure, quiet, chubby girl who gawks at the thought of attention. Slowly learning to proclaim, "Yes I am a big girl and I am beautiful." I didn't need a boy to tell me "you're pretty" to believe it. I needed to hear it from myself. As I got older, I started to see me for me, and I liked who I was becoming. I was doing well in school, naturally funny, easy to talk to, enjoyed singing and writing rap songs, and following my own fashion ideas that made me feel confident but comfortable. Yes, compliments are cool but more meaningful when they are coming from the person who matters most … ME. Undeniable, beautifully crafted in His image, wrong to some right to none. I was learning to accept Ria G for the person she is.

While learning to embrace the exterior side of yourself, the bigger question to ask is who the person is underneath? Pastor TD Jakes said it best, "There is a lot of great advertisements out there, but the product is bad." You can always work on losing weight, changing your hairstyle, fixing your crooked smile, or changing up your wardrobe. But who you are as a person, well let's be honest, you are either "a vibe" or not. Working on our inner selves takes time, commitment, and leaving some people behind for that type of change. The real lesson is learning the value of people, not quantity but quality, recognizing who someone is beyond who they appear to be, including you. Life is short. It's best to spend your time with those who add something to it: more love, more empathy, more intellect, more comedy, more of the good stuff life has to offer that is not materialistic.

Journal Question:

When did you know you were coming into your own style? What or who influenced you? Can you recall a time in your past when someone opened your eyes to see beyond physical appearance? How did that make you feel?

_____

_____

_____

_____

_____

_____

_____

_____

_____

_____

_____

_____

_____

_____

_____

_____

_____

_____

_____

"I found I was more confident when I stopped trying to be someone else's definition of beautiful and started being my own."
—Remington Miller

_____
_____
_____
_____
_____
_____
_____
_____
_____
_____
_____
_____
_____
_____
_____
_____
_____
_____
_____
_____
_____
_____
_____
_____
_____
_____
_____

Chapter 8

Voted in ...
Hurt People Hurt People

Dominique

I was tired of waiting at the library for my mother to pick me up after school. She was always late! You see, I inherited my addiction to retail from my momma. Good ol' Glyn always found a store to stop and shop at before picking me up.

Finally, I was fed up and decided to join the after-school program at the neighborhood church. This was not your ordinary church program. All participants were voted in. On my first day, I was so nervous and feared no one would think I was cool enough to join the group. Then I met David, a fifth grader, and he was sooo cute! He sat down next to me, and we immediately started talking. I was in shock and wondered why or how he noticed me. David looked at me and said, "Don't worry, you have my vote. You're in!"

I later found out he was the most popular boy in camp and whatever he said went. Over the next few months, David and I had a whirlwind elementary romance. We had an unspoken connection. Everyone knew I was his girl, and I loved the attention. At nine I was domesticated, making sure to have his peanut and jelly sandwiches waiting for him with his banana on the side when he got off the school bus daily. I remember the joy and sense of belonging I felt.

The one day I'll never forget was a normal day after school. I made David's sandwich and ran outside to meet him at the bus stop. As he hurried off the bus, frowning, I yelled with a smile on my face, "David, I have your sandwich!" He snatched the sandwich and threw it on the ground and yelled, "Leave me alone, fatty!" My heart sank! I remember my friend Porsha defending me and begging me not to cry. *He's such a jerk*, I thought, devastated. Out of shame and a fear of rejection, I dreaded the thought of being teased or seeing David's face again. So, I did what I did best at that time in my life, I hid. I told my mother I wanted to stop going to the after-school program, with no real explanation. Completely heartbroken, I was too embarrassed to tell anyone how afraid and ashamed I was.

Looking back, I wish I had stood up to David. When we hide, we give people's words power over us. That power runs deep and creates scars that are forever etched in our hearts, building walls of resentment.

In my earlier years, I remember being teased as my weight moved up on the scale, even by some family members and so-called friends. The taunting reinforced the negative beliefs I had about my self-image. When questioned about being teased, I made an excuse or denied it. Yet, I cried in private and begged God to stop the torment. I never allowed others to see the pain I felt from their words and ridicule. I kept it inside, building a fireproof wall of defense rooted in shame and anger.

One incident still sticks out in my mind to this day. Back in my day … I can't believe I said "back in my day." I really am old. Okay, let's get back on topic. We didn't have TikTok, Facebook, Instagram, or social media. We had Jerry Springer and three, four, five, or six-way phone conversations. On this particular day I was on the phone with my elementary crush and two other friends. My crush was being silly as usual and began to crack jokes on everyone. I was hoping he would forget about me, but of course, he didn't! He started talking about my weight and called me "fatty." I laughed it off as usual and felt my heart sink when I heard someone in my house pick up the phone. I immediately got off the phone and ran downstairs.

My sister looked at me with concern and said, "Dominique, are people making fun of you?"

With a confused expression I said, "No, why would you ask me that?"

"I heard someone say—" but I cut her off and yelled, "Fatty! They were talking about someone else!"

"Okay," she said. "Just know real friends won't make fun of you."

I realize that would have been the optimal time to expose my friends and share with her how hurt I was.

As I blossomed into a teen and young adult, I too began to hurt and taunt others with my words, finding myself retaliating against or humiliating those more vulnerable than me. My mind was made up: no one else would hurt or ridicule me ever again. I lived on the defense, not understanding how my words mirrored my own self-thoughts.

Now in adulthood, I am learning that being defensive blocks one's ability to heal or find inner peace. Playing defense forces one to live on the edge, never cultivating the beauty that lies within. You see, confidence is an attitude. Confidence could not care less about the size of your waistline or exterior image. Confidence isn't rooted in how others see you but in how you see yourself!

Reflection:

I don't fully understand why the human brain is wired to fight or flee from pain. My quest to protect myself led me down a path of taunting and hurting others to maintain my defenses. I no longer trusted myself, friends, or the people closest to me. Although I was too embarrassed to tell my sister the truth that day, I do not doubt she knew the truth. I think her love and compassion for me wouldn't allow her to expose my lie.

The adult version of me realizes David may have been suffering himself when he lashed out at me that day. If you know anything about zodiac signs, you understand a Cancer isn't called the crab for nothing! We harp on everything, and man, can we hold a grudge. I have learned the hard way the importance of letting go. Anger, bitterness, and strife eat away at a person, leaving you to wallow in self-pity while the other person has moved on. Do yourself a favor. If you feel like I'm talking to you, please choose forgiveness today. Remember, life is too short to allow anyone to have power over your mind, spirit, and emotions.

We as a people have to do better in teaching our children the importance of empathy and showing compassion toward others. Webster's Dictionary defines empathy as the ability to understand and share the feelings of another. When we possess empathy, we choose our words carefully, and think twice before insulting someone. I believe empathy teaches respect. It's also important to see the strength that lies in being vulnerable. It is okay not to be okay! Not one person is superhuman or without fault. Yet, we try our best to be perfect, which is why so many of us suffer in private. It is acceptable to admit that we are in pain and someone has hurt us. Likewise, it is also okay to apologize when we have hurt someone. It is time to take ownership of our actions. Let's start telling the truth to those we hold close to our hearts and trust. The truth allows us to seek the support and advice we need to heal and move forward. The state of our mental and emotional health depends on our transparency.

Many of my clients find an immediate weight lifted off their shoulders after their first therapy session as well as a profound peace that follows because they have found a safe space to share their stories. I understand how intimidating or unnatural speaking to a therapist can be. Our role as a therapist is to facilitate a conversation and guide an individual toward making a sound decision. This book has allowed me to speak my truth. For years I was afraid to admit I was teased as a child. I associated being teased with weakness. Not understanding, so many of us have carried our wounds in secret. Think about an experience that you have carried with you for years in secret. How did this experience shape you into the person you are today?

I leave you with this. If you can't be honest with anyone else, please be honest with yourself.

Journal Question:

Do you remember the first time you felt rejected? What did that feel like? What did you do to manage those feelings?

_____

_____

_____

_____

_____

_____

_____

_____

_____

_____

_____

_____

_____

_____

_____

_____

_____

_____

_____

_____

"I am no longer willing to pretend that your rejection of
my feelings is anything less than a rejection of me."
—Stephi Wagner

Chapter 9

Lil Kim Taught Me Best

Ria

I n high school you have plenty of pre-adult first time moments. Mine was the day I got my first job at McDonald's off Mayfield Road in South Euclid, Ohio. Mr. Paul, the manager at the time, took a chance on a young and eager ninth grader ready to work. My favorite part of the job was the free meals (dare I say it). I had access to fries, shakes, and finally tried my first Big Mac. It was something always advertised on TV, but I was too embarrassed to ask my mom for one because I was a big girl. I never wanted her to think I was gradually turning into a hungry hippo.

My dad was really proud of me. He cautioned that I should be in no rush to work because I would spend the rest of my life doing it. He realized I had the same hustler spirit and the drive to be an independent young lady. The purple polo-style shirt with the golden arches and tight black khakis delivered a sense of undeniable pride. There were times I spruced up the McDonalds purple polo and visor uniform, draped in my gaudy jewelry stand pieces from Tower City, our downtown city mall: Mickey Mouse rings, silver-esque Nike chains with matching rings, and post earrings that spelled my name down the ear lobe (benefit of a three-letter name).

Earning my own paycheck enhanced my plus-size style while under-standing the value of a dollar and the stores I loved. Learning my body type and what clothing made me most confident was challenging. I was a femme tomboy. Monday through Friday I was confined to a skirt for school during my entire education with the exception of some winter months, we had the option to wear pants. I hated the way I looked in dresses, often comparing myself to a linebacker in a skirt. My calves were muscular, accompanied by broad shoulders, and my big butt often hiked the dress up in the back. I didn't feel feminine at all. Because of my strong build I often wore men's shoes with my school uniform, like low cut Timberlands with designer logo knee-high crew socks. I never wore the expensive uniform blazer my parents purchased. Immediately, I went for the embroidered school logo crew neck sweater. I just felt more comfortable dressing down my dreadful plaid skirt!

More often than not I wore men's designer clothing too: Tommy Hilfiger, DKNY, Polo, and Nautica (jeans, t-shirts, button ups with a white tee underneath, and sweatshirts). Men's jeans (in my opinion) fit me better throughout the thigh area. To appear more "girly," I would buy the men's shirts smaller to accentuate my waist that was always smaller than my lower body. Obviously, this fashion era presented itself before jeggings, skinny jeans or any stretch denim. Seriously, I owned one pair of women's jeans in high school. My notorious light blue jeans were bootcut and faded white in the thighs. I bought them in a size 18 from a fashion store called "Deb," and I held onto them for years. I wore them with feminine tops when I wanted to look really cute for a guy I liked.

I was curvaceous. My mom made me feel ashamed of my derrière, with her constant reminders to pull my skirts or shirts down in the back. But let me tell you, all that shame went out the window when I heard the song "Baby Phat" by De La Soul. The first time I heard the lyrics and saw the video, it confirmed my existence. "No matter how you wear it, girl, it's feminine." Ayyyeee! This song empowered me and my growing coke bottle shape. I realized some girls just have more to offer, and I was one of them. Not everyone will like it, but someone will love it.

My taste in clothing required more money per hour than I earned at McDonalds. I elevated my employment to support my shopping habits. The summer going into junior year, I applied at The Finish Line, a popular tennis shoe store in Euclid Square Mall and got the job! A total game-changer for this teenage girl. Waving goodbye to the golden arches, I was in a completely different league. The obsession for fresh sneaker soles was born, proudly wearing the turquoise polo and tan khakis. Back then you couldn't tell me anything with my thirty percent discount, okay!

Around this same time, my teenage freedom presented itself when I acquired my driver's license . Teenage freedom to drive myself to school, work, friends' houses, the mall, secret missions to see the opposite sex, and parties. That fall, my parents bought me my first car (the "Banana"), an off-yellow two-door 1989 Mercury Topaz with nothing automatic inside and a tape player for cassette tapes. I will never forget my dad asking me if I wanted him to put shiny hubcaps on it. It was "a thing" back then, but I politely passed.

Rides to school or work provided personal time for valuable life tips from Lil' Kim, "All I wanna do is …" I mean, if you know the song, you get my memo (R-rated most definitely). My mom was constantly in my business and rightfully so. Dar wanted to know "who, where, what, and when" anytime I left the house. She was overprotective of her beautiful, curvy, smart, and ready to explore the world daughter. My Mercury Topaz was the sanctuary for personal exploration into ratchet rap music, figuring out boys with my homegirls, learning about love songs, sneaking Glacier Bays and Smirnoff Ice weak alcoholic drinks to DJ Steph Floss high school parties. I became a connoisseur of Lil' Kim, Foxy Brown, Notorious B.I.G., Jay-Z, all of No Limit, Musiq Soulchild, and Faith Evans. Music became second nature to me. For a moment I was inspired to write my own lyrics, fantasizing about hitting the stage with some of my idols. "I'm only 17, a mother's dream, working, getting my own cream …" Obviously, my rap career didn't take off, but it's never too late!

By eleventh and twelfth grade I was discovering my shero independence: establishing my academic road for college, earning my own paychecks, and enjoying typical teenage rides of a lifetime (in and out the car). I talked to older guys because I played the mature role well. Going to an all-girls school made it hard to meet boys my age, so most of the time I met the opposite sex while I worked at the mall. However, the three guys I talked to at the time were not people I would run home and tell my parents about with full excitement: in their 20s, jail records, two had pending court cases, two had baby mama drama, all three lived at home with family, and there was one who was the definition of evil. If we opened the dictionary his picture would be there.

Daytona was attractively built like a football player, cornrows in his hair and dimples in his cheeks. Sammy was slim, tall, dark brown with the waviest hair and the warmest smile. Snag … well … he was older than the other two, a small guy with terrible teeth who worked at the rival shoe store in the mall, Footlocker. I think Snag offered me extra attention, teaching me that men will provide this to get what they want. He never succeeded, and after a while, I got turned off by his smile. Ugh, I just couldn't take it.

With a serious mean streak, just like a Cancerian, Daytona was in the streets. Honestly, I couldn't tell you if he was a Cancer or not, now that I think about it … well, never mind (I never knew his birthday). His street mentality blocked any ability to give me the attention I was used to. I think Daytona saw me as a conquest (I'm going to get this virgin good girl). But he pulled back when I became clingy. You know, calling him back-to-back or just pulling up to his neighborhood, hopping out the car in front of the corner store asking his friends, "Have you seen Daytona?" What the hell was I doing, man? He would invite me to his friend's apartment, where we would 'hang to Netflix' but no full on chill! He probably thought I was a tease and got tired of it, honestly.

The second guy I talked to, Sammy, was a sucker for your girl. He just had too much going on. Fresh out of the city jail, he walked into The Finish Line looking for shoes. We exchanged numbers, and he was in love with me. I tried brushing him off, but he wouldn't let go. I used the "I'm going to college" routine, but he insisted on waiting for me. He was in a back and forth relationship with his son's mom, going in and out of county jail, and his mom hated me. In her defense, she did walk in on us in her back room, not going all the way but it was pretty close. One thing I can never take away from Sammy is that he loved me, but it was just too much at that time. He wanted to "wife" me up, and I just wanted to run off to college and kick it.

Guys from my high school past fueled my self-confidence, permeating the notion, "You may be chubby, but girl, you're IT. And don't let anyone tell you otherwise." I will credit my infamous intuition in the making. Despite being a heavier girl and unable to maintain the typical appearance of most teenagers my age, such as routine acrylic nails and hair styles like salon perfect updos with a swoop, majority of my self-esteem came from holding onto my virginity like it was the key to the city. I knew what guys wanted—SEX, but no one impressed me enough to make that big decision. Majority of the time I was confident about making the right decisions for myself despite typical teen peer pressure. I learned how to follow my own mind, if I'm being totally honest. My mother always taught me (and I found her advice to be true as I got older): "Don't ever sit somewhere uncomfortable. If you don't want to be there, then don't." This small piece of advice goes a long way. When you are making a decision, are you comfortable with it? If the answer is "no," then don't do it.

The "men" I talked to or "dated" (and I use that term loosely), provided attention, but truly were in no position to date anyone their own age: no car, no place of their own and no stability. When you are a teenager, usually you are not able to see people for who they are; you have not lived long enough or experienced much. Luckily, I had enough self-worth to walk away from these men before anything crucial occurred. They offered me attention and that was it. I went to an all-girls high school, so male interactions were slow for me, non-existent. But I was smart enough to see beyond the words they were feeding me: "Girl, me and you are going to be together forever. You are the one." Well, of course they felt that way! I was in a far better position than they were. I was smart, attractive, on my way to college, had my own job, and a car. I mean, how could they think any less of me? Unfortunately for them, I was wise beyond my years, considered myself more of an actions-versus-words type of girl. If someone's actions didn't match up to their words, I never put much thought into them.

Reflection:

For some of us, our teenage years were a rebellious time in our lives, pushing limitations and testing boundaries of those caring for us. Not only are some of us testing the waters of our new freedom like driving or dating; we are experiencing life-altering decisions. Peer pressure can become distracting, and the outcomes of what you decide can go either way. As I became older I realized why my mom was "strict." She cared about me and still does, if not more. I felt like she was constantly in my teenage business (we all thought that). Asking me where I was going and with whom and stated what time she expected me back home. Darlene being strict, asking these questions contributed to the type of teenager I was: responsible enough to consider the consequence of my actions. Not only did I have enough self-worth and love not to fall for the bare minimum words of "men," but I always considered the outcome of my decisions.

This is what I want for you moving forward. Remember your self-worth and love when you are interacting with people. When discussing your plan of action, what is the outcome? Will this be a potentially positive or negative effect on you? Now, let's be honest, there are times when you will not know this answer until you actually try something out. However, the power of intuition is strong and will help you. Trust your first mind, trust your gut. If there is a voice deep down telling you "no, don't do it" or "something doesn't feel right," listen to it. Believe it or not you are smarter than you think. You may not have all the information you need sometimes, and you do not need it to make the right choices.

We grow into our adult selves and reflect on where we've been and where we are. If you can look at yourself in the mirror with a roof over your head, transportation if needed, clothes on your back, taking care of your own, and not asking anyone for a damn dime, consider yourself "doing damn good." If you had someone in your life promoting self-worth, love, and confidence (or teaching you independence or self- sufficiency), thank them. If you had to learn this on your own, you are the real MVP at this thing called life.

However, it is not fair that you had to take on adult responsibilities as a teenager or learn adult lessons the hard way when you should have been worried about homecoming dances. It is not fair that you did not have anyone in your corner telling you how beautiful or handsome you are. You will always be the prize, not for what you look like but for who you are as a person. I want to hug you, and I'm sorry you had to experience what you went through. Your past does NOT define who you are, and this is only a part of your story, not the final chapter. Do not stay tied to your roots from the past. TD Jakes said that!

Journal Question:

Describe the high school phase in your life? If you could change something about it, what would it be? Knowing what you know now, what advice would you give the high school version of you?

_____
_____
_____
_____
_____
_____
_____
_____
_____
_____
_____
_____
_____
_____
_____
_____
_____
_____
_____
_____
_____
_____

"Pay attention to the people that care. Who are always there. Who wants better for you. They're your people."
—Unknown

Chapter 10

Everyone Loves a Sleepover

Dominique

As if middle school isn't hard enough, right? Becoming a teen, puberty, and the introduction to girl drama is a complete subset of life's problems. Seventh grade was a hard transition for me. Separated from my elementary school friends, I was sent to a local Catholic school. I found it extremely hard to fit in and find my place, but finally, I became friends with three other girls. We often hung out in and outside of school. The three of us understood the plight of being slightly thicker than the other girls in school, while our fourth counterpart of this girl quartet was slim and a class favorite. Around this time, I was satisfied with just having a pretty face and long hair.

When I was younger, my mom did not believe in sleepovers. When I got to middle school, I guess she figured I was old enough to protect myself or tell her if I felt unsafe. So, the sleepovers began!

One occasion that sticks out in my head is a sleepover that three of my friends and I had. I took extra precautions when sleeping at the homes of other people. When getting dressed and packing up my clothes, I was careful to cut or remove tags, so no one would know what size clothes I wore.

Have you ever cut tags or found yourself insecure about your dress size? But during this sleepover, I forgot!

Two of my friends were whispering about what size I wore. They laughed and said, "Who knew she was that big!" I acted as if I did not hear them, but I remember feeling embarrassed. My stomach turned with queasiness, so I went to the bathroom to calm down. My friends noticed a change in my mood and demeanor; I was disengaged and quiet for the rest of the evening. I found myself tossing and turning the entire night, replaying their words in my head, unable to sleep. To this day, I wish I would have had the courage to confront them and share how much they hurt me. I would have crawled out of my skin if possible. Sweat dotted my forehead and pain rippled in the pit of my stomach. Throughout the night my discomfort increased. Several thoughts raced through my mind. Was I overreacting, or should I confront my friends? I was tired of being the butt of others' jokes. Was this payback for teasing others in elementary? Lord knows I am not innocent or free of guilt when it comes to teasing or making jokes at the expense of others. I learned to make fun of others to deflect and take the attention off myself. Yes, I understand how this sounds, but sarcasm became my superpower and ultimate defense mechanism. I never wanted to be subjected to the pain and shame of being teased for being a fat kid in elementary. Therefore, I vowed to stick up for myself in middle school, yet I was falling into the same trap. The trap of being weak and silent and feeling both hopeless and helpless.

All my experiences before this had taught me to keep a low profile. Being ashamed and thinking I was 'less than' and putting on the tough-girl facade was my mindset. The truth is I did not have the confidence to stand up for myself on this particular night. I was too vulnerable and unsure of myself, which caused me to enter into several unhealthy friendships over the following years. Subconsciously, I believed I was at the mercy of other people's actions. I was afraid of losing a friend despite how toxic the relationship was.

As an adult, I understand the importance of maintaining healthy and reciprocal relationships in both friendship and intimacy. Now I run from toxicity and value my peace, self-image, and sanity! I am both selective and protective of who I allow to enter my space. Friends are truly the family members you choose. Choose wisely, and remember a true friend loves, supports, and is invested in seeing you become the best version of yourself. True friendship should inspire, challenge, and rally for you.

I am encouraging all people to accept their bodies fearlessly and boldly. To demand and expect healthy reciprocal friendships. You are deserving of love and friendship. Never settle for being less than your best self! Wear your size with confidence and shine. Remember, you are the prize!

This experience stuck with me throughout my adolescence. I found I was not the only tween uncomfortable in her skin. According to an article featured in *Frontiers in Psychology*, appearance-based teasing is a common phenomenon in social interaction, especially in adolescence (2019). The results from this study found that women showed higher impairments in body image, mental health, and lower self-esteem due to being teased. Further proving the lasting effects of ridiculing others based on their differences. This experience coupled with others from my past led to body dysmorphia. The Mayo Clinic defines Body Dysmorphic Disorder as a mental health condition in which you can't stop thinking about one or more perceived defects or flaws in your appearance. I wonder what makes people at such a young age do and say such hurtful things. Is it our life experiences that make us ridicule and demean one another? Is it the daily pressure that women face when watching TV, listening to music, or now the ever-so-daunting presence of social media?

This experience taught me the importance of building each other up as young women. It is important to let people know when they have hurt us, and to be mindful of our actions to avoid inflicting pain on others. Something so minimal caused huge feelings of despair in my thirteen-year-old mind and body. Internalizing the hurtful words of others led to an unhealthy obsession with the imperfections of my body, dreading the thought of trying on clothes in public or looking at my reflection in the mirror. For years I allowed the words of some people to haunt me and shape my interactions with others, thus creating my distorted view of friendship. A view that taught me to sacrifice my feelings and allow people to disrespect me without any fear of retaliation or consequences.

Reflection:

A real friend allows you to be yourself. They don't judge you but instead show their support. What I learned and now realize is I had no reason to be ashamed about my size or of being exposed. We all have flaws or characteristics that we dread anyone shedding light on. Those two whispering behind my back weren't real friends! Yet, I was too afraid to stand up for myself. I thought I needed their acceptance. So I feared being left out and alone. I needed to fit in at the cost of my feelings.

As I became more comfortable with myself, I paid less attention to the number on the scale or on the tag of my clothing. I began to value the attributes that made me a good friend, creative, and special. My love for clothes gave me a newfound freedom and sense of self expression. As people began complimenting me on my sense of style, I received a boost in my self-esteem and confidence. I no longer desired to inflict pain on others to protect myself. I wanted to encourage those around me. Holding my head high, I became an advocate for the underdog. I used my voice to speak for those who were bullied and found themselves feeling the way I once did.

Who can you advocate for? Take a minute to pause, and then ask yourself: Iis there anyone in your life that doesn't have the confidence to speak up for themselves? If yes, why? Let's face it, so many of us allow people to break our spirit because we don't believe we deserve more. We listen to the negative words we tell ourselves and stay in toxic relationships at the expense of our happiness. Today, I refuse to sacrifice myself for anyone. Let me say that again … Anyone! We all deserve to be happy, whole, and at peace with ourselves.

I encourage you to choose you. Let go of any shame or guilt and let the past be the past. Walk in your truth with your head high. Let go of the petty, jealous, and self-absorbed people in your life. I promise you will find another friend circle that welcomes you with open arms. Remember, you're worth it!

Journal Question:

Were you an overweight child, or is there something about your body that you wish you could change? If yes, how did childhood obesity affect you emotionally? Do you still struggle with the hurtful words of others? If yes, in what way?

_____

_____

_____

_____

_____

_____

_____

_____

_____

_____

_____

_____

_____

_____

_____

_____

_____

_____

"The mind remembers the words, but the heart remembers
how it feels. The mind can forget, but the heart never will."
—JM Storm

Chapter 11

Full Off Foolishness

Ria

Finally, I'm free (from my mother)! College was challenging for me in terms of my love life, creating the foundation for my early adult relationships. Freshman year was my true college experience. Partying every weekend (random fraternity parties of all ethnicities); my version of the walk of shame (drinking with my friend Gino from Cleveland who stayed on campus and staying overnight in his dorm to cuddle (we never had sex); doing well in my classes (shout out to my general studies folks); falling in love … all within ten months. I tried avoiding the freshman fifteen, but it was inescapable. Away from home, three meals a day of whatever you pick, endless varieties of beverage machines, and partying late at night, devouring Taco Bell or White Castle food, will pack on pounds. If you didn't have a workout routine or some sense of well-balanced eating, when you returned home for holiday breaks, family or friends noticed. It could be the "surprised" look on people's faces or comments like, "I see you're eating down there" that could spark weight insecurity. My weight gain was not as significant, but I was aware of it and tried working on it. I walked to class and maintained a low carb diet through college, just to maintain my weight (190s to low 200s).

My most successful weight loss story in college happened during fall quarter of sophomore year. I was fresh off the initial trial of the "no-carb" diet I had committed to all summer. Wheeeww!! I got all kinds of compliments from guys and girls saying, "Damn, Ria! Okay, I see you." My mom introduced me to the Atkins diet during the summer after freshman year, eliminating carbohydrates from all meals aiding in rapid weight loss. I focused on "proteins' ' (pork rinds, meats, cheese, eggs and diet Pepsi). Simple enough to follow all summer long. Not old enough to legally drink alcohol, those additional sugars were not an issue. Exercising was easy. I often went to Forest Hills Park or the Patrick Henry school track in my neighborhood to run/walk, do jumping jacks, push-ups, and sit ups for a good hour in the mornings. Morning workouts get your day started in the right direction, ya know! This "Atkins-ish diet" was my permanent meal plan throughout college, keeping my carbohydrate intake at a minimum. I opted to save room for important foods like Chipotle or hot wings from Pizza Hut (the six-piece combo). At the time I was not a big "snacks" person. I saved my calorie intake for my one meal of the day. This is NOT healthy or how you lose weight. My water intake was nonexistent at the time. I was more of a "diet soda anything" girl because of the no sugar content, rationalizing the health factor.

Boys came and went, and eventually, I stumbled across Patrick: a tall, heavy-set, medium tan, loudmouth from this small town in Ohio. He wore braids, always had a sucker in his mouth, and was the campus herbal supplier. I fell completely in love. He was a little rough around the edges, but he had to be smart. I met him on campus, right? Wheeew, I knew he was the one. I wish I could tell you Patrick and I had this whirlwind college romance, king and queen of campus who dominated the academic circuit. We were not. People knew we were together and that's it.

The reality of my Bearcat love was completely opposite: It was the first love rollercoaster from love hell that I experienced. Brought me down just as quickly as it took me up. In the beginning it was mutual physical attraction that brought us together. I went into my relationship with Patrick feeling cute, confident, and not overthinking much of anything really. During college I was your typical, financially struggling college student but always maintained my own affordable style. I wore the best Old Navy and Ralph Lauren Polo outlet clothes that I could afford and fit me at the time. My shoe game was decent: standard all white Nike Air Force 1s, a pair of 504 gray New Balance, a few pair of Timberlands, and random old school Adidas I loved. I was doing fairly well to be your average broke college kid. Patrick would call me his "Italian Mami" which sounds really dumb saying it out loud. My mother is African American and Italian, so that was his reasoning for the nickname. Patrick never expressed an issue with my size. The more slender girls that he flirted with made me feel insecure. On the outside looking in you would have thought he had an issue with my size, not sure if he chose not to say it directly or out loud. Instead, he opted to "innocently" flirt with girls who were slightly or significantly smaller than me. I felt like I was in competition. Thinking back to this bothers me even more. He needed my help to keep up appearances with everyone else on campus! Whenever my school refund check came, Patrick always hit me with a "Do you think you can get me this from Footlocker" question. The nerve!

Patrick thought he was slick nonetheless, a true master manipulator. He would get defensive quickly when he was wrong. No matter what we argued about—it was my fault. Patrick was quick to accuse me of talking to other guys behind his back, guys from my extracurricular groups, or if we visited the mall in my hometown and I saw a guy I knew in general. The starry-eyed college love we shared was R&B singer Khelani's "Toxic." I would humiliate myself in the halls of our dorm, curse him out, and become physical toward him. I learned the person constantly accusing you of dirt is the dirtiest. Finding condoms in his jean's pockets or travel bag that I let him borrow, girls eyeing me on campus. Patrick knew exactly how to push me over the edge by not answering my calls or his door after an argument. Jealousy motivated us from different sides: his being manipulation and mine being insecurity. It was never equal. I paid for majority of our dates though we both worked. There was always an excuse, "Oh, I had to give my brother money … Oh, I had to do this … Oh, I had to do that …" He worked part time at United Parcel Service (UPS), and I worked somewhat part time hours at The Finish Line shoe store at the local mall in Cincinnati, not too far from campus. By then I was a junior in college, and we both had our own cars and attended classes full time. But during my nursing program I was also a full-time Resident Advisor to help pay for college. My academic plate was full. One would think Patrick would acknowledge this and say, "Wow, I need to step my game up," or "Wow, I need to treat her like gold."

NOPE. I take responsibility for not demanding more or tolerating what he gave, the bare minimum.

I don't know if I stayed with Patrick because I did not want to finish college single and worry about having sex with someone new? Or, if I knew I was breaking things off with him when senior year ended, so I just said, "F**k it, let's just ride this relationship out."

Spring break of senior year I was attending my first set of professional nurse interviews, preparing for nursing examination boards and college graduation. I did a survey of where Patrick and I were in the relationship department. Over the last five years together, I reviewed our accomplishments as individuals, and they did not align. He had taken a break from school, moved off campus with his homeboy Steve attempting to make it into the rap industry (to my knowledge he did not), and continued to work part time at UPS. That was it. There was no forward movement in his life. I always worked part time during college and maintained my Resident Advisor position until graduation. I was selected to participate in a paid nursing co-op program senior year sponsored by my BSN program; completed my nursing program; received graduate nurse job offers; prepared for my nursing boards. It was clear we were not on the same page with starting our post-college lives. Not long after graduation I broke things off with him upon returning home to Cleveland, Ohio. That door never reopened. By the end of our Bearcat Love Story it became clear I learned to become comfortable (which is never good) in fear of not wanting to be alone. I worked too hard academically, preparing myself for a future career, to settle romantically. I deserved better than what Patrick had to offer. I was not better than him, but I realized my worth and he never did. After five years, he was still in the same place when we met: hanging out on campus, flirting with other girls, and working part time at UPS.

Reflection:

It is crazy how we find ourselves in relationships at different points in life questioning ourselves in the end. Like, how dare you, you super deluxe dope creation by God sit there and allow someone to make you feel like you aren't "good enough!" The hell? Baby you ARE, and do not allow anyone make you think or feel different again. If they could not see the light shining around you, let them admire the shadow it leaves as you exit their life. Why? Because they were not ready to receive your presence anyway.

After my relationship ended with Patrick, I realized it was okay. My college relationship was not the storybook love most people talk about. The problem is people go into common life experiences like high school or college and run the risk of disappointment when it does not turn out like the storybook happy ending. It is okay if it does not turn out picture perfect. You will recover. Allow this time in your life to be a learning lesson if nothing else, the good and bad, uncomfortable and unknowing parts. That is what life will be anyway. It is not your assignment to coach people into wanting the same things as you. They have to want them just as much, especially when the tools to be successful are at their disposal. If your relationship taught you something to take with you, the growing pains may have been worth the while. I walked away realizing my future was too bright to be blinded by what I thought was "love." I spent the last five years preparing for adulthood, and I deserved to put myself first.

You should also remember putting your needs and wants first when you have no attachments to someone. When you find yourself single and free, allow your wings to expand and explore wherever the wind takes you! This is your moment to do so. We try to follow this road map of life: high school graduation, college, fall in love, get married, etc. But sometimes the "traditional" path is not for everyone, and that is okay too. God's plan for you is tailor made, so sit back, be patient, and enjoy the ride.

Journal Question:

Do you recall your first serious relationship? Would you describe this as a healthy relationship or not? Did this relationship change you for the better or worse? If so, let's talk about it.

_____

_____

_____

_____

_____

_____

_____

_____

_____

_____

_____

_____

_____

_____

_____

_____

_____

_____

_____

_____

"You deserve someone who lets you glow
in every way you need to."
—Nikita Gill

Chapter 12

Friend Zoned

Dominique

I remember looking at the other girls in my elementary classes, thinking, *If only I could be beautiful like them. They are skinny, and all the boys look at them in awe.* These girls had the attention of one boy especially: Brandon. I had the biggest crush on Brandon but never thought he would like someone like me. He came to my house on the weekends, introduced me to his family, and was the best companion a girl could have. However, he made fun of my weight and teased me in front of our classmates. He often called me fat or said I was big and made jokes referencing my size during lunch. Drawing attention to me and making me the butt of everyone's joke. I would shrug off his jokes and try my best to change the topic as quickly as possible. Typical school-boy behavior—hit and bully the girls you like. Seriously … we really need to change school-age interactions between girls and boys.

Mentally wounded, I hid my pain and continued to be his friend. I fantasized about being skinny and what Brandon would think of me then. Rejection and shyness taught me how to friend-zone myself because I looked different. I also knew I would never share with Brandon that I had a crush on him or thought he was cute. Honestly, I was afraid of showing interest in anyone that I liked or found attractive. At a young age, I learned a friend could not be rejected or humiliated if their feelings remained a secret. So I did just that and continued to lay low and behind the scenes. Laying low was safe. I found a sense of security in knowing that I kept my deepest, darkest desires and secrets to myself. I feared expressing my feelings to Brandon and losing our friendship or being viewed as weak by him or our friend group. I had to keep up my image of the cool fat friend. I had to appear strong, because that is the mask I had worn for so long. As a child I learned to live a double life and portray myself as happy while I was internally suffering. I am not naive and know that almost every child across the world has endured some form of bullying. Despite the nature and frequency of bullying, children need to know that it is okay to ask for help. Fortunately, most schools have a zero-tolerance approach to bullying. These policies and level of awareness did not exist in the early '90s, and I am not sure if I would have exposed my perpetrator.

My puppy love for Brandon transcended the hurt I endured at his hands. I was able to overlook the taunting and remained hopelessly loyal to him. As an adult I understand how dysfunctional this sounds. I associated love with feelings of pain and protected my offender. I get it, but we were children and my failure to speak up played a part in his actions toward me. I wonder if he would have apologized or stopped teasing me, if I shared how his comments affected me. Knowing the fun, loving person he was, I truly believe he would have felt some remorse.

Although silent, I recognize the level of resilience I exhibited. I learned the healing power of laughter, writing, and found I had a passion for learning. Because I was fat, I strove to excel academically and take an interest in my education. I became the teacher's helper and stayed back from lunch to grade papers. This saved me from the torment I often experienced at the lunch table and boosted my confidence by giving me a sense of belonging. I now identify as being pretty and smart, which began to overshadow being overweight as I got older.

Fast forward. I arrived at high school and finally began to find my way. Yes, I might have been on the thicker side, but I thought, at least I'm put together. I regained my sense of self-acceptance. Although I was still insecure, my newfound love for who I was becoming took precedence.

I began to see I had a good sense of humor. Academically, I continued to perform well and tried new things. I think the support of my two best friends at the time thrust me into this new reality. The three of us struggled with our weight and identified with one another. We affectionately called ourselves "The Three Musketeers!" Our friendship helped me regain self-confidence. I will forever be grateful to the other two women in this trio for the part they played in my life.

Brandon and I remained friends throughout our youth. I remember a conversation we had in high school when he began to share how he'd always had a crush on me in elementary. I was stunned! Uncertain how to respond or react to his confession, I felt my heart beating fast, and I sat silently in the room. I could not bring myself to tell him the truth about my feelings for him, too. I was afraid of being laughed at. Secretly, I wondered if he was playing a cruel joke on me. I remember looking at him with a blank stare, refusing to show any emotion. I continued to lay low behind my first wall of defense, the "friend zone," kicking myself for not being honest. I thought, *Dominique, why?* This was my chance to bare my soul and finally be seen. I remember him looking at me, waiting for a response, and I remained stuck like a deer in headlights. I don't think I ever truly acknowledged his comment but laughed and quickly changed the subject. You see, I reverted to our childhood interactions. Deflect when I felt like my back was up against the wall or in an uncomfortable situation.

As I moved on to the next topic, his demeanor quickly changed. His voice began to crack and the usual confidence he exuded slowly diminished. For the first time he appeared unsure of himself. Although uncomfortable, for the first time I held the power in our relationship. I realized he shared the feelings I had toward him. Somehow I finally felt justified in my emotions.

Yet the thought of being seen was more dreadful than feeling dismissed.

Reflection:

Unfortunately, learning to keep my feelings under lock and key prevented me from being the best version of myself. I was too afraid to walk in a crowd or step out of my comfort zone. I did not believe guys noticed me. *How could they like me?* I thought. Now looking back, I see that I did not like myself.

I was always waiting to lose weight to shoot my shot—not realizing all the shots I missed.

To this day, I still regret not being honest with Brandon. What did I really have to lose? Sure, I would have had to let my defenses down and put myself out there to tell my truth, but I believe it's better to be honest than hide behind a lie.

I learned that being shy and aloof had been two of my biggest downfalls in all my relationships. I have walked around with an "I don't care attitude" while I'm crying or dying to be noticed by people of interest or my partner. People, I am here to tell you, this is completely foolish! Life is all about taking risks, and I learned the most about my character in times of failure. Plain and simple, rejection is a part of life.

None of us like it, but rejection builds resilience. In many cases, it acts as a safety mechanism to protect us from ourselves. We often think we know what is best for us and go into relationships blindly. Today, I am thankful for every letdown and failure I have experienced. Because of it, I am a little stronger, wiser, and more cautious. Embrace the bumps and bruises that have made you who you are. Bet on yourself! Talk to the classmate or coworker that you have a crush on. Initiate a conversation based on your interests. Know that you are talented and beautiful with a lot to offer. Yes, sharing your feelings is scary, but you may be pleasantly surprised. Many of our fears are based on a lie or negative thought. Such as: "I am not smart or attractive." I have found that failure is the antecedent to success. Each heartbreak, toxic friendship, and mistake are all a part of your story. A story that may help someone else discover self-love.

Journal Question:

Have you ever found yourself in the friend zone? If yes, why were you afraid to share your real feelings?

_____

_____

_____

_____

_____

_____

_____

_____

_____

_____

_____

_____

_____

_____

_____

_____

_____

_____

_____

_____

"Do not tame the wolf inside you just because you've met someone who doesn't have the courage to handle you."
—Belle Estreller

_____
_____
_____
_____
_____
_____
_____
_____
_____
_____
_____
_____
_____
_____
_____
_____
_____
_____
_____
_____
_____
_____
_____
_____
_____
_____
_____
_____

Chapter 13

The Roaring Twenties

Ria

One of my most accomplished times in life has been college graduation. A set of credentials behind my name, "BSN" (Bachelor of Science in Nursing), and I secured the first nursing position I applied for and wanted by my early twenties. A medical surgical telemetry nurse job with one of Cleveland's well-known hospital systems. I was preparing to start my nurse intern position as a pre- Registered Nurse where I would learn my role until I passed my state test. It was a paid position with the hospital making $15.50/hour while working side by side with a nurse preceptor. Trust me that was big money back then! I was back home in Cleveland with my friends, catching up on what I missed with them while I was in Cincinnati; going out to whatever clubs were "poppin'" (the place to go) at the time: The Moda on West 25th Street, The Millenium downtown, The Cocktail on Superior Avenue, and all of West 6th on the weekends. Things were looking up post-breakup with Patrick. This is also the time in my life where my past (AC from elementary) revisited, and it was least expected.

Somehow I found myself in the arms of my elementary school crush, AC. A simple phone call rekindled our connection. AC and I casually kept in touch over the years but not strong enough to maintain life details. By this time, I knew he had two kids by the same woman and was working as a barber with one of his older brothers in a hairshop. He looked exactly the same, with the exception of some facial hair, cheeks still big and round with that cheesy smile. I wish I could recall our first adult date. I do remember going out to dinner on one of our earlier dates to a restaurant on Euclid Avenue near Case Western Reserve University, it had a grown and sexy vibe to it. It was time to pay and in my naiveté, I offered to go half. AC looked at me and said, "No woman of mine will go 50/50. I will always pay." I just knew this was it, such a 180-degree change from dating Patrick. How could it not? Elementary school puppy love maturing into something more!

AC and I went to parties and clubs together, and we enjoyed plenty of typical date nights. We ventured on our first vacation cruise, and he threw me a huge surprise birthday party one year. He was crazy about me, and I was crazy about him. We really enjoyed one another as adults. I even loved bringing him lunch to work. Cancerians are affectionate with people they are attracted to, that was never our issue. When we got along he made me feel beautiful and secure. AC could be very loving and sweet beyond our physical connection; it was visible in public and private. People would see us out and just say, "You two are sooo cute." I never questioned his loyalty toward me in terms of other women or felt embarrassed about my size. During our courtship I was a size 18, but I was working out and feeling genuinely good about myself. Also, I had my first nursing job earning an adult paycheck and affording luxuries of self-care. Simple pleasures like maintaining my eyebrows, hair, and nails in addition to upgrading my wardrobe instantly boosted my confidence.

However, the adult version of our puppy love affair was more than I bargained for, leaving me emotionally bankrupt. AC pulled a fast one on me. Not only did he leave me emotionally bankrupt, but I lost a couple dollars along the way. But when you're in the midst of something, your decision making can be swayed. In my case it was love and the desire to build a life with AC. We got an apartment together, and I was adamant on having ALL NEW everything. Though he was a fellow Cancerian, he did not have the same passion in this department, so it was "on me" to furnish our home as I saw fit. He was fine with his old dusty mattress from home and I refused. This was the start of our downfall. AC was furious about the new mattress I bought to replace the weathered one he brought from home, I just couldn't do it. I did not like the idea of sleeping on a bed in our new home that AC had romanced a bunch of bodies on, nah. To show his disapproval, that man slept on our new bed less than ten times in that apartment! Talk about petty. He either fell asleep on the couch (I could not stand it) or slept in the second bedroom.

When our relationship was bad, it was a damn disaster—like National Weather Alert status. Cancerians can easily detach from people. We can turn cold when we are really upset or feel like you've done us wrong; we can become mean and just retreat into our shell when we do not want to be bothered by anyone. AC was a true champion at this between the two of us. I had not quite mastered this tactic in a relationship with the opposite sex. In all honesty, we did not see eye to eye on most things: It disturbed me how he handled things toward his children's mother. He was the type of man who would stop doing things for his kids if he got into it with their mom. *What kind of shit is that?* I thought. He stopped picking his daughter up from school when he got into it with their mom once. There was no way in hell I entertained the thought of having a child with him. Another example, he had an older brother who would often spend the night after bar/club hopping (he had his own place). It bothered me because this was the same brother who had an issue with me staying over-night at their house before we got our own place! The difference between AC and me in the midst of war was, AC was a sharpshooter, and I was a novice to the range. Though he loved me and my curves during the good times, you would have thought I sold his social security number for a credit card scam during the bad ones.

One Christmas after an argument, AC left me sobbing uncontrollably on the floor in the second bedroom of our modest apartment. Distraught, I recall trying to pull my s**t together to head over to my parents' house, drinking a bottle of Smirnoff Ice while listening to one of R&B's greatest, Anthony Hamilton. Damn, AC could be so damn evil. It seemed as if I was always last to know when we were on the "outs." He would be upset over something from days ago, and out of nowhere decide not to speak to me days later for days at a time. This happened more often than not. During these moments, AC would talk on the phone and laugh with whomever he was speaking with and purposely ignore me. Cancerians are moody, but you never knew which AC you were waking up to that day, surprising you like your menstrual cycle at work.

We had a hell of a run, but I was tapped out. Cancerian love is pure at heart, raw emotion at best, and addictive if not careful. You love the good times, smiles, laughs, and affection you two share. You know deep down in your heart you both love each other but are incapable of doing this correctly. Ultimately, you never hear your partner out. I remember swearing off Cancerian men after AC, it was not negative attributes alone of our twinning horoscope that created a ruckus between us. It was the lack of understanding toward each other in the relationship. Things I learned from my AC love story:

- A partner should make you feel comfortable speaking your peace without fearing retaliation.
- Disagreements should be had respectfully, even if you agree to disagree.
- Strive for healthy mutual give and take (financially, emotionally, physically, etc.).
- Observe the relationships people have with their immediate family.
- Pay close attention to how a person treats their child(ren) and the parent of their child(ren) in general.

If you pay attention to these things early on, it may save you a headache and/or heartache later. I carried these lessons with me into my future as a gauge with other men who crossed my path.

Reflection:

One of the key elements of a healthy relationship is "communication," and you will find this in any relationship book or online source. The communication in our relationship was terrible: lacking and unhealthy. Dialogue requires a messenger and receiver. You know, two or more people having a discussion to resolve an issue or taking part in conversation (Oxford Dictionary, 2022). AC and I were two people talking but never listening to each other. We both were quick to respond in the moment for the sake of our feelings toward the matter. When two people can have a disagreement or misunderstanding but respectfully discuss how each person feels, you're on the right track to healthy problem-solving. You two must give each other an opportunity to speak freely and hear each other out. Hopefully, you two can move forward after deciding on a solution that makes you both comfortable. If there is no solution that can be agreed upon, you two should at least be willing to respect your difference of opinions and continue to move forward the best way possible.

Honestly, I found my voice after this breakup; it was liberating. Like taking off your bra after a long day. I promised myself not to hold my tongue with the next man or any other for that matter. Moving forward, I promised to let people know what I do and do NOT like in relationships. In the "talking" or "early dating" stage, I tell people immediately my basic relationship "do's and don'ts: don't lie, especially when it's obvious, just be honest. If the person I'm dating has a child(ren), do not speak to me like I'm one of them (I really don't do well with that). Another big one for me is don't tell me you are going to do something for me and not follow through, big or small. On a lighter note, I enjoy mild public displays of affection (hand holding or the off guard back rub). Whether they hear it or not is on them, but the way I look at it, "Hey, don't say I never told you." Please take my advice on this: when you start dating someone, let them know up front your "do's and don'ts." This should avoid the likelihood of one of you two being caught off guard three, six months, or a year into your relationship.

Speaking up for myself has always been a challenge. Yes, because for years I conditioned myself to stay low key, keep quiet, and not draw attention to being a "big girl." But what I am learning is my feelings ARE valid. The way something affects me IS important. So baby, speak now and do not disrupt your peace. Do not allow someone to dismiss or downplay your emotions, certainly not yourself! A relationship should add safety and security to your space of being. Both of you should be pouring into each other's cup with communication and various displays of love language. We need to understand in relationships when someone is sharing their feelings, as a partner it is our responsibility to hear them though we may not understand or agree. In turn, you must feel safe to speak your mind or say what's on your heart. But remember, it is not what you say but how you say it. You will always attract more bees with honey, right? So when you want someone to hear you out, try to collect your thoughts and calm your emotions. I know this can be hard as hell. But cursing, name calling, and just pure back and forth disrespect will make you "feel good" in the moment. But ask yourself will it solve anything if that is truly the intent?

Journal Question:

Have you ever rediscovered your voice after a breakup? What did you learn about yourself once the relationship was over?

_____

_____

_____

_____

_____

_____

_____

_____

_____

_____

_____

_____

_____

_____

_____

_____

_____

_____

_____

_____

_____

_____

"Love people enough to tell them the truth and respect
them enough to trust that they can handle it."
—Iyanla Vanzant

Chapter 14

Not the Right Boys

Dominique

Boy, oh, boys! I found myself never liking the ones who liked me and vice versa.

Please know I was never willing to settle for the boy who liked me if the feelings were not mutual. I had enough confidence to know I was *not* a charity case. I would rather fade into the background than be with a guy I was settling for. I started telling myself, "When you lose weight, the guys you like will like you too."

My best friend in the ninth grade was a serial dater by the age of fourteen. She was in love with the idea of love and was determined to find her happily ever after before we turned eighteen. Which often left me feeling like the third wheel during many of our weekend adventures. After months of pleading with me and trying to convince me to go on a blind date with her boyfriend's cousin, I folded and gave in. He was fair-skinned with red hair, freckles, and overweight. He was from Alabama and preferred that the girls he dated be plus-size.

Despite being charmed by his interest in me, I couldn't deny that the spark between us was missing. My friend couldn't understand why I didn't like him. To be honest, I am not sure if I was turned off by his weight, or if I gave him a real chance. At that age, I was more concerned with what other people thought of me. I may have projected my feelings onto him, which prevented us from forming a relationship. He was kind, attentive, and genuinely interested in me. Yet, I couldn't look past his exterior. I was still stuck in the mindset of what our society and culture perceive as attractive. I like to think that I am pretty open-minded, but I fell into the trap of judging a book by its cover instead of getting to know the inner person. Many of us are carrying years of baggage and judgment that has spilled into our relationships with others. It is time to identify the events and words that led to these emotions and negative self-talk. Begin to speak positivity and life back into yourself. It is true that when we know better, we do better, but that takes honesty and courage.

Why did I think I had to change or change others to find love? I look back and see those were NOT encouraging words to myself. And here we are, feeding into the horrible lie ... something was wrong with me just being me. Today, I would tell young Dominique, "Be patient, because true love doesn't require you to change."

Middle Man

It was the middle of my junior year in high school, and I had my wit and a solid friend group. For the first time, I didn't question if I belonged. Attending an all-girl high school was trying at times. My friends and I loved to go to basketball games and mingle with the opposite sex. This particular night we were at a basketball game at St. Peter Chanel High School. My friends Rachel, Sonia, and I were a trio that hung out inside and outside of school. Rachel was pretty, popular, athletic, and a free spirit. Sonia was pretty, thin, and known for being overly judgmental. We all shared a love for sarcasm and enjoyed the freedom driving gave us.

During the game, Rachel went to sit with a guy she was talking to during halftime. I remember sitting off to the side, with no expectation of hooking up with anyone. I was content with sitting with my friends and never fully experiencing the "boy crazy" phase of my youth. Rachel came running back to her seat and said, "Dominique, everyone kept talking about how cool you were, and they think you're pretty too." I looked at her confused because I often thought I was invisible. I acted as if I didn't care and brushed off her comment with a chuckle. She looked at me and told me how silly I was, and then went on to the next topic. Little did she know how her words replayed in my mind. As small as it may seem, I realized I was not invisible, and my weight did not count me out as I thought it would.

A few months went by, and Sonia asked me to ride with her over to the house of a guy she was interested in. Sonia was notorious for dragging me to the new dude of the week's house, and of course, like a good friend, I went. I remember entering the house and noticing this was a setup. Sonia disappeared, and there I was, alone with her new beau's friend, Max. Max was fine, but he had a reputation for being a little too free sexually for my taste.

Max and I talked for a while, and he began to move in. As he moved in closer, I stepped back and continued the conversation. I remember thinking, *I know he doesn't think I'm going to sleep with him!* It didn't take Max long to realize he wasn't going to get to first, second, and definitely not third base with me. I was sitting with my thoughts when Sonia came out of the bathroom fixing her hair. She asked if I was ready, and we left. In the car, she asked if Max had tried anything, and I told her no, to avoid the conversation, but to his defense he didn't step out of line. I remember the confusion on her face when I told her I wasn't interested.

Reflection:

True love accepts you the way you are. As John Legend sings, "… All of Your Imperfections." Be you, just the way you are, unapologetically you. Knowing that you are ENOUGH! High school to me was a time of self-discovery, trial, and error. I found my identity. I had a new friend group and was outgoing. I no longer walked in the shadows of others and felt confident in my wit and new social circle. During this time, I learned that I had a talent for giving advice. I became the voice of reason for most of my friends. Often I was viewed as a prude for making conscious decisions and for my inexperience with the male counterpart. Many of my friends continued to set me up with their boyfriends' friends or drag me to the seediest environments for their next hookup. I remained a loyal and nonjudgmental friend. Soon I realized that all my friends, those fat and skinny, were like me. We were all stumbling through our adolescence, making mistakes and trying to find our place in this world. We all witnessed and engaged in the typical girl drama, looking for someone to love and accept us.

High school was hard enough, and I knew then I didn't want a reputation. Yes, I craved male attention, but I was not willing to have sex with just anyone to be liked. I wanted to be loved and realized sex was sacred to me and not to be shared with just anyone. My religious beliefs made me feel guilty for having sex before marriage, and I wasn't willing to add another notch to my belt and risk feeling stupid again. My relationship with Ishmael scarred me. I did not want to go through another heartbreak or give someone else an opportunity to play with my emotions or laugh at me with their friends.

Bottom line, at the end of the day, we have to live with the consequences of our decisions, good or bad. You should not have to lower your standards or be disrespected to receive attention or have a relationship. Don't be afraid to be yourself. Conduct a self inventory prior to dating. Think about what you offer or bring to the table in a relationship. Write down a list of non-negotiables, which are characteristics you are not willing to compromise for anyone. Be aware of your value system.

Journal Question:

What is important to you? Do you value education, religion, financial security, etc.? How do you want to be treated in your current or next relationship?

_____

_____

_____

_____

_____

_____

_____

_____

_____

_____

_____

_____

_____

_____

_____

_____

_____

_____

_____

_____

_____

_____

_____

"You really are good enough, pretty enough, and strong enough."
—Al Carraway

Chapter 15

I'm Not Your "Break" Bitch

Ria

There were some short-lived romances after AC, but the one I choose to highlight is Byron. Byron was a familiar face from my junior high years. We did not attend the same school, but we knew the same people from the neighborhood. He was always cool, comedic, and had a playful energy. He was absolutely my type, you know: medium height, glistening brown skin, and a big white smile that could light up a room. Facebook may be the reason Byron and I reconnected. An innocent friend request upgraded our interaction to innocent inbox messages, and the ultimate exchange of phone numbers for an in-person "remember when ..." conversation. Of course it was nice at the beginning (like always). Standard movie dates, going to the gym together, hanging out at his place. I loved drinking the solid staple of Barefoot Moscato overlooking the lake on his upper Lakeshore Boulevard apartment balcony in Eastlake. I started liking Byron ... a lot. Though I had ended things with AC a few weeks ago, I just refused to idle in my singleness. I enjoyed being in the company of the opposite sex. My long-term relationship in college made it difficult for me to be alone for long, as I mentioned before. Besides, Byron was gainfully employed, no kids, own place. I mean, sounds like the single girl direction to move forward in love, right?

Ummmm, *no*. This turned out to be completely opposite of love. I will take ownership for the majority of his comfort during our "talking"/dating phase. In the beginning, he would call at any time of the day, and I would go running out to Lakeshore Boulevard, allowing myself to appear too "thirsty" or "pressed" to be around him. It did not matter if I was meeting him at the gym or picking him up because he had worked all night. I was there within twenty minutes, okay! Splitting the cost on our outings sometimes, I mean, why not? It's platonic. We were not exclusively dating each other (rolling my eyes) … Ugh! This sounds awful just saying it out loud! A part of me wanted to prove how supportive I could be as a mate if given the opportunity. You know, more of it was showing how down-to-earth and understanding I could be too. Playing my position as a real "Ride or Die" for someone who did not think enough of me to exclusively date, let alone consider for a monogamous relationship … just dumb.

Somewhere between our casual hanging outs that were definitely Netflix and Chill moments (sex), Byron became comfy—and quickly. I was about 230 pounds at the time. I always went to the gym and worked out to sustain my physical appearance. I carried my size pretty well in the "right places" like buttocks, hips, and thighs. However, Byron started size-shaming me! Can you believe that? We worked out together, true, so it wasn't like my effort wasn't there. But I was not starving myself to be a size two. I ate meals and good ones like shrimp and scampi pasta! He said something along the line of "If you were a size so-and-so you would be perfect …" I will never forget how he made me feel—like I was good enough to have sex with but not good enough to have a serious relationship because of my size. From that comment forward, I knew this would be nothing more than a physical friendship, no matter if he "acted" like a boyfriend behind closed doors, he was friend zoned in my book.

I had already eliminated any romantic feelings for Byron, strictly using the situation for what it was: sex. At some point, our physical encounters became boring, you know. Something to do but nothing I looked forward to anymore. I recall lying there in his bed one afternoon, thinking, *B***h, this ain't even worth it—my time, his actions, or the energy.* Later in our talking phase, he got laid off, lost his Dodge Magnum, and was damn near kicked out of his apartment. He thought I was a "good neighbor" type of woman.

After sitting in the ER one evening with him for an earache, sore throat, or something minor, I thought, *Naahhh, I'm good, and I wish you better*. It was the realization of giving 100 percent for someone who more than likely wouldn't give two percent for me. And at the time, well, he really couldn't. But his treatment toward me had become such a turn-off, I knew where this was going. Nowhere. Now his chips were down, and he thought he could lean on The Good Neighbor B***h? Abso-f***ing-lutely NOT! I ended our "friendship" after a brief two or three months of gym, Netflix and Chill and never looked back. I stopped taking his calls and blocked him from contacting me (I will block someone in a minute, baby. I don't believe in useless connections). I noticed he follows me on an old Instagram account, and I will leave it there for now. I deleted what I really wanted to say at the end of this chapter because I'm focusing on my growth.

Reflection:

Some men are idiots straight up, and you will waste your time overanalyzing the situation when it goes wrong because there are endless what-if's. Is it something I did? Am I the problem? What if the timing was off? NO. Just stop. It's not you ... it happened for a reason when it was supposed to. The problem is people's callousness. The nerve of someone to criticize you for your jean size while they're losing a place to piss in. Make it make sense for me. Thinking about the feelings you had for them and the support you provided with more to give, only to feel ridiculed for your waistline? Oh, okay! It's a damn shame; his mom really liked me, too. Byron taught me the importance of the phrase, "It's all good, luv, enjoy." I've never been the type of person to kick a person while they are down, but the audacity to treat me like an option made it easy for me to walk away. Byron did not deserve my time, attention, or support, so why bother to extend any of those luxuries to him when he may have needed them most? This is what you need to ask if you are in a similar situation. Does this person deserve the gift of my time, attention, and support? If they do, by all means, provide it for them. If not, "Stop!" Do not allow another minute to pass where you are giving them access to your luxuries.

I could continue to hold a grudge toward Byron, but there is no point in that. He is simply another male in my life who reminded me that I can add to any table, but I would be a fool to settle when I have my own table, chairs, and place settings at the house! What everyone needs to realize is the importance of identifying personal boundaries. Write a set of guidelines for yourself that you are not willing to bend. These are your personal values that can help people know how you expect to be treated. I went with the flow while hanging out with Byron, often agreeing to things I was not okay with, like doing most of the driving on our dates. Even if your situation is platonic or titleless, do not allow your needs to fall by the wayside. Verbalize them, and if the other person involved does not respect them, re-evaluate if it's worth your time.

Behavior like Byron's and how I decide to deal with certain situations contribute to my Great Wall of Ria, making it harder for the next love interest. Surely, I needed to be a better judge of character, and honestly, my standards were, well … non-existent. I gave anyone a chance if they appeared to be cool. A familiar face was a sense of comfort, so the Welcome Home mat was ready at the door.

Trust me on this: Set your standards high in what you want from a mate when dating to avoid wasting your time in the long run. For example, if punctuality is important to you, tell people that when arranging times for dates. Let them know how it makes you feel when someone is constantly late for plans. I can't promise you that you will have perfect relationships, but I would like to help you avoid meaningless ones if possible. You want to spend your time and energy with people who pour into your life's cup, not subtract from it. People who actually listen to your wants and needs; follow through with their actions; teach you new things; bounce ideas off each other and show support; consider how something would make you feel. Creating high standards and boundaries should help you experience quality relationships with people, leaving more positive memories than not. It does not matter what your family or friends say or what negative vibes try to cloud your light, you are worth everything you deserve from the universe.

Journal Question:

Is there someone you've dated who you wish you wouldn't have? If so, why? What did you learn from this experience?

_____

_____

_____

_____

_____

_____

_____

_____

_____

_____

_____

_____

_____

_____

_____

_____

_____

_____

_____

_____

_____

_____

_____

"Sometimes your heart needs more time to
accept what your mind already knows."
—Unknown

Chapter 16

Most Sacred Gift

Dominique

L et's rewind. It was my sophomore year of high school. I wanted to be like all the other girls and explore being young, dumb, and in love. I just wanted someone to notice me, like me, and most of all, love me. What started as a simple phone call led to a whirlwind of puppy love and infatuation.

Ishmael and I were introduced by a friend of mine in high school who was dating his best friend. I remember our first conversation like it was yesterday; our young love blossomed over the phone. When he asked what I looked like, I described myself as "thick." I avoided meeting him in person for months, afraid of being rejected or judged by the first boy I allowed myself to connect and build a bond with. We immediately clicked on an emotional level, and I was not willing to lose our love if he didn't approve of or was turned off by my weight.

I held out until I ran out of excuses, and it was finally time to meet in person. I remember wearing heels and layers to appear smaller. As we met in the Tower City food court, I thought, *This is it, I can't turn back now!* Ishmael and I sat down and talked. He was handsome, sweet, and seemed just as interested in me face-to-face. He offered me his last piece of Taco

Bell, and I was sold! From that moment forward, all I saw was "Ishmael." I was in over my head, and he became my drug of choice for years to come.

We laughed, texted (on our pager), and called each other throughout the school day. I was finally a "normal" teen! I had a boyfriend. After dating on and off for almost two years, Ishmael did not seem as interested as he was in the beginning of our relationship. The phone calls began to slow down, and our once fun-filled conversations became dry. In a state of panic, I began to think of ways to put the spark back into our young romance. I thought having sex would bring us closer and make him interested in me again.

Boy, was I wrong. I remember sneaking away and giving him my most precious gift, my virginity—exposing a life lesson experienced by many: Sex comes with heartbreak and complications. After awarding him my most prized possession, the texts and all-night pillow talk stopped. I was played, bamboozled, and fooled! I tried my hardest to reignite our spark. I mean, if he didn't want me, who would?

My insecurities lied to me once again! I was back at square one, invisible and undesirable to the opposite sex. I accepted less than I was worth, in a conquest for his love and approval. Waiting for him to pick me or see that I was worthy of his love. I permitted my hurt to take me down a long road of pain and deception. My young heart soon realized I was not the only girl Ishmael was dating. I tried to entice him with sex, to steal a moment of his time. Yet he continued to show his lack of interest time and time again. He would profess his love and go missing for days and weeks without a call.

One incident that sticks out in my mind occurred in the spring of our senior year in high school. Ishmael reassured me that I was the only girl for him, and he no longer wanted to hurt or betray my trust. Naive and eager to rekindle our love, I believed and accepted him with open arms. During our teenage years, both Ishamel and I loved to go out to the local teen clubs in our area. This particular night we planned to meet at the Cotton Club. I walked in with my friends and immediately noticed Ishmael in an argument with another female who was crying. Without thinking, I walked up to Ishmael and said hello and introduced myself. Ishmael, stunned, darted for the nearest exit. The young lady who was with him introduced herself as Karen. She was heavier than I was and appeared just as hurt and confused. Immediately she said she was Ishmael's girlfriend and just found out he was cheating on her. Mortified, I told her I was his girlfriend too. She looked at me and said, "Oh, are you his Catholic school good girl? He told me he loved you." Unfortunately, this became a central theme in our relationship. Ishmael was a serial cheater, and I became addicted to the toxicity. I prided myself on being the "one" he loved. Not realizing, he didn't love me either. Yet, I felt comfort in knowing he told his other women about me. I tricked myself into thinking I was different, smarter, or more special than the other women he was with. Soon, our toxic romance led to an unplanned teenage pregnancy at the age of nineteen. I was devastated and knew I was in over my head. But I was determined not to be another statistic or looked upon as a failure.

Reflection:

Listen, young ladies and young men, your virginity is a sacred gift that should not be taken for granted. Take your time! I allowed my distorted view of self to rush me into this life-changing decision. My lack of self-esteem and battle with weight led me to believe I was unattractive and undesirable. I was desperate for Ishmael's acceptance. Everyone is in a rush to grow up until they make one decision that leads to a lifetime of drama and heartache. Teenage pregnancies, diseases, and financial hardship are not part of a life anyone dreams of. I rushed into a sexual relationship to maintain a relationship that ultimately fell apart. I overlooked the red flags that presented themselves at the beginning of our courtship. Because I was unwilling to see the harsh reality those around me attempted to shield me from, I was forced to grow up prematurely. When you take things slow, you allow yourself time to get to know the real person you are dating instead of their representative. Lust, infatuation, and living on cloud nine are normal feelings. However, when the spark is out, you want to like the person you are lying next to.

Look at any successful relationship. You can tell they have a solid foundation rooted in friendship. Your partner must be your friend, and not the person you only call to Netflix and Chill. Listen to that small, still voice on the inside. I believe all women possess a level of intuition that is often silenced because we choose to ignore it. Pay attention to the signs. Actions truly do speak louder than words. A person who values your time will call you and invite you out on dates. They will be honest and respect your time. A man who only calls you to have sex doesn't want to display his affection in public, introduce you to his family or friends, or isn't dependable is not looking for a long-term relationship. If he doesn't answer his phone in front of you, turns his phone off when you're together, or you can't reach him at night, he may be hiding something. You should not have to look through phone records, read texts, or direct messages. Trust your gut. Do not settle for less, you deserve more. Trust is earned!

"As we are liberated from our own fear, our
presence automatically liberates others."
—Nelson Mandela

Journal Question:

Did you rush into sex? Do you feel your first sexual encounter was influenced by your partner, or were you ready?

_____

_____

_____

_____

_____

_____

_____

_____

_____

_____

_____

_____

_____

_____

_____

_____

_____

_____

_____

_____

"Sometimes it lasts in love, but sometimes it hurts instead."
—Adele

Chapter 17

Damn, I Thought
She was a Dude

———

Ria

Somewhere between my ex, "32," and the start of my brief nursing travel career, my first assignment landed me on the East Coast. A small town outside of Philadelphia in Reading, Pennsylvania. The paychecks were nothing to brag about in comparison to today's travel nurse rates. I made about $650 per week (I know you're gasping). Now I will inform you that my position at the time was in a stroke rehabilitative medicine unit not an intensive care unit or an emergency room. My background is medical surgical nursing so I had to take what was available for my skill set at the time. The apartment was sweet as hell, another reason why the paycheck was not as much. Agencies would pay you more if you had your own housing, if not they would provide the housing for you, and it was usually pretty nice. It was in a gated community with a new workout facility, business center, swimming pool, and newly remodeled living spaces.

I worked the evening shift and during my thirteen-week stint I met Briana. Hella cool; I mean, she lived through a soul beyond her time. Imagine this combination: Nasir "Nas" Jones and Erykah Badu in one with a hint of Gandhi. At the time Briana stood about five foot four, slender in frame, flawless 360-degree hair waves, and whatever cologne she wore always lingered. Casually dressed in her scrub attire layered with her thermal long-sleeves, bubble vests and fitted caps.

We became friendly, initially talking about work and the common observations on the unit. We were the minority, aside from the unit secretary who was a beautiful Puerto Rican woman and a younger male nursing assistant who was adorable and hardworking, also Puerto Rican. Our venting about work graduated to hanging out after work like trips to the mall and local restaurants to grab a drink. Eventually I found myself establishing closeness with the same sex differently than just "friendly." I admitted to her, "For the longest time I thought you were a guy working here!" She laughed and didn't take it personally. Our friendship grew into something more than expected, very new and uncharted in my book. It was the first time I was "talking" to someone of the same sex. Briana was very special to me. We took obnoxiously cute photos together, went to social gatherings side by side. She even bought me my *Sex and the City* DVD series for Christmas that year. It was the only thing I wanted. I damn near cried … Finally, someone (besides my best friend TJ) gave me a gift I actually wanted. Briana was someone who looked at me for who I was on the inside. She admired my mind and spirit. This was something I was not used to. Sure, she thought I was attractive physically. When we kissed there was no denying the passion between us, but we connected beyond the physical connection too. We had real conversations about everything: clothing, music, poetry, family relationships, life experiences, tattoos, travel, work, college, etc. Though she was more slender than I was, I didn't feel embarrassed around her about my size. I'm sure I slid a joke or two in there at some point about myself at certain times, to feel at ease and she paid those jokes no attention. She thought I was perfect as is.

At the time, I wasn't sure what was going to happen. I was just going with our flow … we were into each other. Briana gave me genuine compliments and affection; she would email me poetry, and she paid attention to detail. She knew what to do without being told or encouraged to do so. She was an empath herself and picked up on things naturally. Briana deserved honesty. She was too down-to-earth to have anything less, at least from me. I let her know my intentions throughout our time together. She loved me. I loved her too, but genuinely as a friend. In a perfect world, we would've moved to a cool ass condominium in a major city like Philadelphia or San Diego, adopted one or two kids, and lived a dope life. But during one of our closer moments, it was confirmed that I am not lesbian, and I prefer men. Still, I have always appreciated her vulnerability with me and her immense sense of care.

Over time we tried to remain friends and stay in touch. Realistically, it was just hard. A part of me felt guilty for not feeling the exact same way she did toward me. We had random periods of time where we kept in touch strong for a few weeks, and then it would be nothing for weeks or months. Our reconnecting over the phone was spent sharing relationship stories and offering love advice to each other. I remained supportive of her relationship decisions, though one of her girlfriends blocked our communication for months. Briana was younger than me, and she always dated older women. I was not upset about the situation with her girlfriend at the time it happened. I figured she needed to find her way. Majority of us have been there before. Dating someone that just "ain't right" for us, meaning the person is affecting our growth in some shape or fashion or hindering our financial or emotional well-being. Although I could appreciate the ups and downs of her relationship, after a while, the friendship felt one-sided. She changed numbers a lot and kept going missing in action on social media. It became too much to keep up with. I had gotten to a point in life where my friendships needed to be consistent, and ours just wasn't. I never held that against her. She could have called me out of the blue on any day and seven times out of ten I would've smiled ear-to-ear to see her name flash across my phone screen. Depending on where I was and what I was into. Whenever we finally did talk after a while, we usually did so for a solid forty-five minutes. But losing touch with people for whatever reason, is not necessarily connected to a fallout or feud, it's just life.

Reflection:

Some people come into your life for a season. I feel these connections you share with people are life lessons, both positive and negative. Let's start from the root, friendships are defined as a relationship between people who like each other and enjoy each other's company (Oxford Dictionary, 2022). Now, what draws you in closer to someone are common interests, values, beliefs, and the ability to be yourself around this person. When you connect with someone, you just know. The friendship is effortless, easy. Time can pass, and you two can pick up right where you left off. But friendship is also a two-way street requiring effort from both parties to call, text, email, and make an effort to plan outings. People get busy with school, work, relationships, families, or personal matters. Keeping in touch with everyone on their call log or friend roster is not as important, unless you are someone's "go to" or best friend. Hell, sometimes besties take breaks in between for a day or two. The point is both parties in the friendship must plant equal seeds and be committed to watering those seeds for the garden to grow.

As you grow older, you will learn some friendships will last a lifetime and some are seasonal and that is okay. The shorter "ships" you have are hopefully pleasant, but nonetheless should be a teaching lesson. Hopefully, you learn to appreciate each other for who you are and value the time spent in your season. If you lose touch, or don't speak as much, it happens but depends on the people involved. Some of us can disconnect and rekindle months or years later like no time has passed at all. If you are fortunate, you two will be able to air out any grievances too. Clear any awkward air if there is any and continue to move forward with catching up like no time has passed by at all. You will not find this with everybody. It happens naturally, so when it does cherish these people near or from afar.

When Briana reads this, I want her to know I am forever grateful for her spirit during our season. I hold nothing against her. It is commendable on her part to attempt to maintain a friendship over the years. People change, much like the Cleveland, Ohio weather, so I will always wish her well in life and love. She helped me realize what I deserve in a mate and how I should be celebrated.

Briana, one of my golden gems, I pray the woman who finds you celebrates you and gives you the love you bring to people all day long.

Journal Question:

Can you recall connecting with someone out of your comfort zone but made you feel at home? What about this person attracted you to them? Are you still in contact with this person? Why or why not?

_____

_____

_____

_____

_____

_____

_____

_____

_____

_____

_____

_____

_____

_____

_____

_____

_____

_____

_____

_____

"You are the finest, loveliest, tenderest and most beautiful person
I have ever known—and even that is an understatement."
—F. Scott Fitzgerald

Chapter 18

Not Thin Enough

Dominique

Toward the end of my freshman year in college, I was losing weight intentionally. I made a pact with God and my roommates and decided enough was enough. I was tired of being overweight. I felt my weight made me invisible to the boys I like, and I was fed up. I no longer wanted to be overlooked. I wanted to feel desired and seen. College gave me the freedom to recreate myself and begin a new journey toward self-discovery. I exercised three days a week, didn't eat after five p.m., and denounced all chips, juice, and sweets. The pounds melted away quickly. I was young and committed to the skinny image of myself that I daydreamed about. Entering the summer of freshman year, people began to take notice, both male and female. I thought to myself, "I did it! I am no longer being seen as fat or judged." Often I was asked about my weight loss secret, as if I had a new magic trick that everyone wanted to learn. My friends began commenting on how small I was and compared my shape to theirs. It seemed that for the first time I was seen as their equal, as opposed to their pretty, fat friend.

When sophomore year started in the fall, I had a new strut. I had lost a total of forty pounds and was receiving new male attention. I was wearing my arms out and felt seen for the first time. I even found the courage to pass on a message to a guy I had a crush on. Do not get too excited, though. I later found out I wasn't his type. I guess he said I "wasn't quite skinny enough." Jerk. I remember feeling devastated. *Here we go again*, I thought. I began to get down on myself and think all my hard work was in vain. I thought that no matter what, I would never be the right size.

The feelings of shame crept back in. I found myself settling for a familiar relationship that was toxic yet accepting—my high school sweetheart, Ishmael. I now see that although I lost the physical weight, I didn't do the emotional work to heal the scars of being teased or rejected during my childhood and adolescence. I figured Ishmael was a safe choice, and I knew I would be more than good enough for him. You see, Ishmael never judged or put me down. He saw me for me. Through that transparency, he also saw my insecurities. He realized I didn't think highly of myself and would accept less than I deserved, amplifying my fear of being discarded or never finding someone else who would love or accept me like him. Ishmael preyed on me and other women who were unsure of their worth. He often told me I would never find someone to love me like him.

And you know what? He wasn't lying. I would never find someone else to humiliate or take advantage of me again. Thankfully!

Reflection:

I allowed those negative thoughts to haunt me for sooo long. Listening to the lies we tell ourselves is dangerous. Trust me, true love is healthy and does not take advantage of our shortcomings. I learned that love builds us up and promotes self-love. Love doesn't intentionally hurt or cause pain. Love is pure and is not selfish, but selfless. The dictionary defines love as an intense feeling of deep affection. I feel we confuse this sense of deep affection or admiration in most relationships. Love at times can be disloyal, disappointing, and ultimately heartbreaking. Rejection is a hard pill to swallow. It is easy to internalize those feelings and allow them to block our ability to take risks.

I had to do the hard work to heal and face the demons of my past head on. This meant I had to stop lying to myself and admit that I was hurting as a result of my past. I had it all wrong. I wanted to be normal, but truly everyone's definition of normal is different. The act of being normal cannot be defined by your weight, possessions, economic or relationship status. Yet too often, we place ourselves in a box and beat ourselves up when we do not measure up to society's view of what is normal or socially accepted.

I learned that my journey is different from my family, friends, colleagues, and the surrounding world and that's okay. I found myself journaling, praying, leaning on close friends, reading books on relationships and spirituality to develop a new sense of identity. Understanding how God sees me and loves me unconditionally, coupled with the heartbreak and challenges others faced gave me hope. I believed that I too could triumph over the obstacles I faced. Healing is truly a choice. We must first identify and admit that we are broken, and then we must accept that we need support to aid in the process. Whether you find that support in prayer, friends, therapy, books, podcasts, or family, allow those who love you to rally around and build you up. There is a reason beauty is found in ashes. Sometimes we must go through the fire to find the beauty of who we are. My healing journey developed my purpose. I learned that my story can encourage those who have faced similar struggles, whether relating to their weight, love, or other areas of their lives.

Today, take a chance on you. Take the necessary risk to become the person you have envisioned. Where would any successful person be without the rejections they experienced? Failure is expected. The key, in the words of Donnie McClurkin, is how you get up. Get up and try again! Every day is a gift to start over and bet on you.

IT'S JUST PHAT, BABY

Journal Question:

Have you conquered one of your biggest fears and failed or felt rejected by others?

_____

_____

_____

_____

_____

_____

_____

_____

_____

_____

_____

_____

_____

_____

_____

_____

_____

_____

_____

_____

_____

_____

"… Sometimes fear does not subside, and you must do it afraid."
—Elisabeth Elliot

Chapter 19

Sign Me Up

Ria

Optimistic about jumping into my early thirties, I reminisced about my time on the East Coast and settled back into my hometown. There I met Mitch. Although I've been plus-size my entire life, I have never been a stranger to boot camps and gyms. In college, my best friend Ja'Marie introduced me to the workout lifestyle when our crew was preparing for Spring Bling in Miami, Florida. I did not have the money to go, but I joined their "Fit for Miami" mission. We started going to our campus gym after class together, and eventually I became comfortable going alone.

The gym was always a source of inspiration, admiring my slender classmates on the treadmill or learning yoga ball exercises from fit girl, Melanie. Repeatedly I thought, *"Next summer is going to be my time,"* which meant: "I will be skinny by then, so the world better be ready." That never happened, but still, I always welcomed fitness with open arms. Throwing on my infamous baggy, navy blue Timberland joggers, an old Ralph Lauren Polo T-shirt from high school paired with some old Nike sneakers, I was ready with my Walkman CD player and mix CD from Datpiff (a common music site one would go to for free music downloads) to get a good workout in!

Random: Do **not** feel pressured to dress a certain way for the gym unless **you want to for yourself**. I seldom look cute when I'm headed to workout. Why? My focus is simple: workout and sweat hard. Personally, I feel completely comfortable in baggy sweats, a t-shirt, and a random dad cap putting in work: running, lifting, and doing my thing. Trust me, people may approach you either way (very annoying sometimes) leggings and bra top or baggy sweats and white tee. But if you look unapproachable, more than likely they will not approach you anyway (that's what I've been told). Yet, if you receive compliments or smiles from other gym patrons, receive them nicely, babes, and focus on YOU.

The local gym I attended at the time was decent. It was slightly out of the way, but I didn't mind the drive. I went often, becoming friendly with one of the attendants, a messy, middle-aged man always running his mouth and talking to any woman who walked in the door. A light brown, heavyset guy who was cool when he didn't talk sooo much! He never tried to approach me, just made general conversation, so he did not bother me much. Actually, he did his job well and persuaded me into personal training sessions. I admit I was vulnerable. Officially done with my ex-boyfriend "32" after a quick trip down "maybe we can try this again" detour, I was dedicated to refocusing my energy on myself.

My first session was a weekday, and it was good! Mitch appeared to be serious about helping me with my fitness goal. I wanted to lose about fifty pounds. That first day he pushed me hard. He came off as somewhat tough (no facial expressions). Mitch was in good shape: solid arms, legs, and a strong back. He wore square, dark-framed glasses with a clean fade haircut, but I also noticed he smiled a lot toward the end of the workout. Maybe he noticed how hard I was willing to work, or admired my enthusiasm?

I was speaking with him at the desk, looking at the schedule for our next session, when out of nowhere, he asked me out. I thought it was a joke. He had just worked me to no end on the gym floor, low-key yelled at me, and witnessed my real weight on the scale. I laughed and said, "Whaaat!" Y'all know your girl Ri! Oh, free spirit Ri took him up on his offer. Real smart move. You know the Arthur cartoon meme when he balls his fists ... that's me t y p i n g right now.

My relationship with Mitch preoccupied my early thirties. We ventured out locally, having the standard dates but some outside of the normal ones too. I was simple to please in the dating area. Give me a break, okay? My last relationship with my ex, "32" didn't offer much scenery outside of bar and grille style restaurants and the movies. Mitch suggested our first date location, the new aquarium. I thought, *Wow, taking initiative!* Over time, our friendship flourished. We did everything together, and he was the first guy in my adult life who talked with me about everything in life: career, hopes, fears, even silly, not-so-serious topics. I will admit we did have some good laughs; he would always end the laugh by calling me "baby," paired with a big grin. Over time, we met families and friends, worked out together, and eventually we started going to church too. Funny, I never reached my goal weight, and he spiraled into an interesting journey himself later in the relationship.

Mitch said something to me early on in our courtship though, and it stuck. It was said early enough where I should have promptly disconnected the call and followed up with a "classy" Cancerian text. Picture this: I am on a work assignment sitting on the park bench behind my hotel in New Jersey, minding my business. I participated in a call with Mitch that goes, "If you were a size ten, I'd marry you today." Whaaaat? I can't remember how weddings or marriage became a part of the conversation. Like … the nerve of this dude. His physique was not flawless, not an etched abdominal muscle in sight. But okay, his confidence goes off.

I remember making the most of my time while living in Secaucus, New Jersey, during my travel assignment at the beginning of my "talking phase" with Mitch. Mostly out of boredom, I remember turning up the workouts. I went to this little gym, all red and yellow inside. Every day I took the train from Jersey into Manhattan for work. I walked from Penn Station to my hospital on 34th and 1st, maintaining another trim adult version of myself. The excitement of a more slender physique drove me to Old Navy every weekend. By the time I left Jersey, I had skinny jeans for every color of the rainbow.

My assignment ended in New York prematurely due to Hurricane Sandy, so I headed back home for good, still talking to Mitch. I started working two full-time jobs with two off days every fourteen days. I tried keeping up with the schedules (including the gym), but I loved watching my money pile up in my bank account even more. So working out fell by the wayside.

The adult weight gain kicked in quickly. I was eating whatever to keep me going from one job to the next, and it showed, discovering my addiction to McDonald's mocha frappes. Eventually I walked away from one job to get my physical self together. The decision was hard to make but it was necessary. My relationship with Mitch was over by this point, with no second act for consideration. Enough had transpired between us, leaving my resentment toward him heavy. I found myself reliving a Byron part 2 situation, except Mitch was my actual boyfriend. We were on two different pages: I was focused on my career, and he was finding himself. I did NOT have the time.

I know you're thinking, *Damn girl, you seem like you hold grudges*. Well, I do. It's not the healthiest thing. However, it formed my self-defense. Mitch and I chartered some rocky waters toward the end, handling an adult situation poorly in my book. Mitch did not make me feel confident in his ability to provide stability, at the time he lacked maturity. I did not feel comfortable with his ability to properly co-parent to my standard if we did not work out in the end. I exercised my right as a woman, end of story.

Somewhere I lost myself and the relationship ended ugly. There were difficult decisions made during our time together. When it was time to follow through, I was alone dealing with emotional consequences. After being the primary driver in the relationship, paying for the majority of the dates due to his early thirty crisis, his decision to pursue college full-time and dare not work, and ghosting me on the day I needed him most ... BYE. The final months between us revealed who he was, in my opinion. He became heavily involved in his church, and I supported him. However, his church placed him on a pedestal, admiring a man who was far from the person I knew. An a*****e putting on a façade as if he had his shit together, knowing damn well ... You get the point.

After the breakup talks, back and forth texts, I was done. Mitch had the nerve to randomly text me a picture of a ring he'd bought for our engagement. Baby, the only thing going through my mind was, "Big girls need big diamonds, and I'm no size ten, soooo ..." Let's discuss this, okay. I had big hands with big curves. I refused to settle, especially when I'd been riding with your ass. Besides, the engagement ring felt desperate and not genuine. It was just "off."

Mitch will still send an out-of-the-sky text at minimum once a year to check in. "Hey, friend, how are you?" Over the years, I've replied with simple pleasantries asking about his family, nothing serious. He is the last person I want to send mixed messages to. I stopped talking to him for an extended period after our breakup, blocked his number and changed gyms. Over time, I forgave Mitch and I unblocked him. His texts were simple and to the point so I did not feel uneasy about the brief exchanges. When you have a clear mind, you're able to follow your intuition when the past revisits you: Should I respond to this message? Is this message or call out of genuine concern? Be careful if you still have romantic feelings for this person. A simple "hey stranger" call or text can easily re-open a door that should not be opened.

Reflection:

Mitch, like Byron, left a lasting impression on me: I'm not skinny enough for a real long-lasting commitment, or I would be perfect if I was smaller. I've considered myself confident, about fifty percent of my life leaning more toward self-assuredness than not. But was I? Mitch did not have a leg to stand on during our time together. He was equally flawed, yet I was the one who had room for improvement? I decided to abstain from dating, relationships, comfortships, and sex—*period*. I sat back, concluding I'd given too much energy, time, and self to unworthy dicks (a few I didn't bother to mention, but they know who they are).

I had spent too much of my adult life settling for guys who showed some interest, some time, and much criticism. My time alone was well spent: back in the gym (a new one), time with friends, and memorable much needed girls trips.

#MemorialDayWeekendMiami. I *lived* that weekend. My best partner in crime, Lil' Tee (she is shorter than me and we argue about this constantly) and I still visit our Fontainebleau memories; it was that good.

Ria's Advice (from a friend years ago)
"Learn to be alone."
—Shay

It was time to seriously reflect on my love life after the Mitch pre-midlife crisis. Nevertheless, I made it through with the support of my mom and close friends. After our breakup I was single for months, a first for me and it was needed. I made a mental list of expectations for my next mate during my alone time, some non-negotiables. I didn't have a timeline for my abstinence from men. I figured when it felt right, I would know.

It took years of heartache, drama, situation scares, and tears to figure this out: you should learn who you are and what you want before entering a partnership with someone else. My six-month love life hiatus taught me how to pleasure myself, make a non-negotiables list, and focus my time on things I enjoy like girls' nights out and vacations. I re-learned myself, and now I value alone time. I spent years running to people when they called, bending my personal rules to accommodate their b******t and wasted time I can't get back. These people didn't even teach me anything beneficial, financially or professionally! It's not like I was dealing with established entrepreneurs, prominent physicians, or lawyers who were putting me on to the game that would help me. Even worse, hell, I can kick my own ass after thinking about the men from my past.

Start surrounding yourself with like-minded people, people who can teach you something for your personal, professional, or financial gain. Start connecting with people who value you as a person. Pay attention if the person provides what you want from a significant other before too much time passes you by. If it does not work out romantically, you can at least walk away with a nice investment portfolio or new set of connections. Do you hear what I'm saying?

Journal Question:

Can you recall dating someone who was hypercritical of everyone except themselves? How long did this relationship last for you, and what was the breaking point if it did not last?

_____

_____

_____

_____

_____

_____

_____

_____

_____

_____

_____

_____

_____

_____

_____

_____

_____

_____

_____

_____

"I'm not sorry for wanting what I deserve ... and
I'm not afraid to walk away to find it."
—R.H. Sin

Chapter 20

The Familiar is Fatal

Dominique

Let's go back to the summer of 2003. It was the summer after my freshman year of college, and I was receiving male attention from every direction. I loved my new body and variety of choices in retail that weren't available in plus-size clothing. I was no longer limited by my size or the stores I could shop in. I was excited to go shopping with my skinny friends, no longer embarrassed by my size or the thought of being criticized. Yet, I was itching for that old feeling. I could not shake my first love, Ishmael. I had become addicted to the familiarity of dysfunction. You would think I would have gotten tired of the cheating, lying, and crying, but I became accustomed to the drama. I missed Ishmael and wanted him to see my new look.

I waited until his birthday to make my appearance. As I got out of the car, he looked at me with bucked eyes and said, "Did you get taller!" I laughed and said, "No, I finally lost my baby weight." He smiled. And just like that, we were back in love.

Ishmael was charming in a sneaky kind of way. He knew how to prey on the weak and use a woman's flaws to his advantage. Vividly, he saw the truth behind my weight loss—the mask I hid behind daily, seeking approval and love. He showered me with affection while we were together but failed to be a man of his word. He would make promises with no intent to follow through. Disappear for days without a call. I knew in my heart he wasn't faithful, but I was afraid to let him go. I would hear rumors of other girls, but I tricked myself into thinking it was untrue.

I remember walking into his mother's living room and seeing professional pictures he had taken with another woman. I tried not to stare or draw attention to the picture, but I was devastated. "Who is she?" I asked Ishmael, and he told me she was his ex who was obsessed with him. I wanted to believe him, but I knew it wasn't true. Sooo … I decided to do what I did best and start my investigation. Within a few hours, I knew her name, the high school she graduated from, and her place of employment. After digging and a couple of days of research, I found I wasn't being cheated on but was, in fact, the person he was cheating with. I didn't confront Ishmael with this new intel. Instead, I decided to get even!

You see, I had met Jamie at the Spy Bar earlier that summer. He was handsome, with a sexy muscular build. I found myself coming out of my shell and tired of second-guessing myself. No longer did I feel the need to hide and found freedom in reciprocating my interest in Jamie. He was three years older and a former high school football player. We danced all night, and I was sold. Jamie and I exchanged phone numbers and began to talk on the phone daily. He made me feel safe, and I forgot about Ishmael. I even thought he could be the one, but then the signs began to surface. I noticed he carried large amounts of cash and a handgun. At nineteen I was naïve, but I knew something wasn't right.

Turns out, Jamie failed to mention he had recently gotten out of jail and sold drugs. I knew early on I was not a "ride or die" type of woman, so I chose to place our newfound romance on hold. Jamie was not thrilled by the distance between us, and yet another failed relationship led me back into Ishmael's arms.

Reflection:

I thought, like so many, that jumping into another relationship or getting revenge was the best way to heal from a breakup. I quickly learned that was not the case. My relationship with Jamie was a temporary distraction. Even though I was not thrilled by his criminal background, I would have walked away for less; Jamie's lifestyle scared me. I did not want to risk my freedom or be caught in the crossfire associated with his criminal activity. I missed Ishmael and was looking for an excuse to run back to him. Although toxic, I was used to the drama that came with Ishmael. Looking back, I realize I was not free from fault in our relationship. I wanted Ishmael to define my self-worth. Because I was codependent and obsessed with an idea of what I thought love was. A big part of my identity was dependent on how he viewed me. We misused each other. We were broken and found security in our ability to run back to each other. I knew he would always take me back, even if that meant I was sharing him with someone else. I turned a blind eye to his cheating at times, telling myself I didn't want a future with him. He was not my top pick or first choice for a male suitor. Yet, the idea of meeting someone new was daunting. I knew the baggage and the heartbreak that came from our relationship. That familiarity became my crutch. I chose to settle to avoid rejection and the disappointment of a failed relationship with a new male counterpart. I know how that sounds, and you may ask, who settles at nineteen?

I don't think I realized I was settling for less than I deserved. I was chasing the fairytale—the teenage Romeo and Juliet love affair many of us get tricked into thinking can be our reality. I thought if I gave him what he needed and met every demand, I would earn his loyalty.

It took me a decade to realize you cannot buy love or respect. Ishmael often told me he was not good enough for me. But I would argue and assure him that he was more than enough. I now understand that he saw what I couldn't at the time. He realized he was not ready or willing to love me the way I needed, which required him to be faithful, honest, and sincere.

Too often, we allow our hearts to think for us. We overlook the warning signs that our mate is showing. Listen to your gut and to your significant other. Ishmael told me he would never be able to meet my expectations or love me, and he was right.

Ladies, let's stop wasting our time and start listening! Pay close attention to who or what a person tells you they are. I have found that men who told me they weren't cheaters or liars, were indeed just that. Get to know the people who are in their inner circle. How do they treat the people closest to them? Ask about their childhood and previous relationships. How do they handle conflict or cope with challenging situations? We are all creatures of habit and rarely change our routine or behaviors.

Journal Question:

What do you think of the phrase "The familiar is fatal?" Have you found yourself running back to an unhealthy relationship?

_____

_____

_____

_____

_____

_____

_____

_____

_____

_____

_____

_____

_____

_____

_____

_____

_____

_____

_____

_____

"You have to learn to get up from the table
when love is no longer being served."
—Nina Simone

Chapter 21

'Fireworks'... It Ain't Even the 4th of July

Ria

My Finish Line days groomed me to develop an obsession with tennis shoes, all brands, styles, and colors. I am an equal opportunity consumer of sneakers. I popped into Footlocker one evening after my school nurse shift, looking for work shoes. Did I need some ... probably not. I just wanted to see what was out there. Nothing impressed me at Richmond Mall's Footlocker, but the salesman was helpful, a real talker. Attempting to sell me insoles that I had no desire to buy. He was good at his job, very convincing. Our conversation changed lanes, and we talked about our careers and goals. I didn't think much of it at the time. His demeanor was friendly but professional (you know, he didn't try to get my phone number). That night, I drove away thinking about our conversation and admiring how driven he appeared to be.

Post the Mitch mess and into my abstinence, I came across Footlocker's (Kevin) Instagram on the explorer page. Mitch and I were over. There was zero interest on my end to start anything new with someone. I was enjoying my newfound alone time. Thinking about a shoe plug for all the Jordan re-releases dropping, I started following Kevin on social media (no big deal).

141

He followed back, which is normal, and we started liking each other's pictures, nothing major. One day he posted a picture of himself in his Footlocker shirt and fresh haircut with a swirl part. I gave it a second view and sent him a message directly. Gently paying him a compliment but leaving it open for interpretation. Not long after that direct message, we had our first date at a popular soul food restaurant in the Shaker Heights area of town.

I wanted to end the date immediately. Kevin was overly confident, giving me "I'm the man" vibes. It was a complete turnoff. I remember laughing to myself the entire time thinking, *He can't be serious.* Yet, I can't even say it was our first and final date, because five years later, we were engaged to be married.

He was not perfect; there was a time I wanted to relocate and forget he existed. We parted ways briefly, came back to love, and parted ways again. Hitting speed bumps, skipping around "do not pass go," and almost crossed the finish line through miscommunication, misinterpretations, mistrust, and qualms of a long-distance relationship. I think Kevin "loved" me for me, though, twenty pounds lighter or twenty pounds heavier, and I watched him morph into the man he was determined to be. Our way of approaching mutual goals was off, but I will say we were both determined for what we wanted. The relationship forced me to look at my inner self while we made attempts to work through our issues. Don't get me wrong, we had amazing moments. Hell, he was the only man I've ever worn a plus-size two-piece around and felt comfortable in my own skin.

When I was with him, I didn't question if I'm too fat for this or that. My only concerns were, "How's my hair and do my nails look good?" Please understand, I had those "God, I'm fat today" moments when your best pair of skinny jeans are not working in your favor. Those days, just grab the boyfriend fit and keep going. In his eyes, I'm sure he thought he did his best to support me. He survived my unexpected big hair chop around 2016 listening to me cry over the departure of my natural inches. He definitely was not as emotionally comforting in the moment as I would have liked.

Let's be clear, he was not an emotional buff, so I conditioned myself not to be upset over his reactions in comparison to mine. Trust me, for a true Cancerian, it is the most difficult thing to do. We wear our emotions on our forehead—damn the sleeve—and it can be overwhelming for someone who is not as emotional. But now that I think about it … you know what—never mind—that is an entirely different book in itself. People who lack the ability to empathize or show emotion, baby, take note of that.

Reflection:

I wasn't searching for him. He showed up unexpectedly with this charming smile, good looks, warm disposition, a hundred jobs (okay, about two or three, hell who knows, definitely more than one though), and two beautiful kids. Kevin had the ability to make his heart appear as if it was in the right place through acts of service and gift giving and that won me over.

You know, we really don't know what the outcome will be when we meet people. There can be an initial vibe of "oh no, this isn't going anywhere" to being happily ever after—well, until you aren't. Maybe we need to pay more attention to our instincts from the beginning. At first, we don't know what's connected to people when we meet them: their past and present, the type of baggage they bring with them. We all have our stuff though: debt, vices, family drama, work issues, legal problems, or parenting concerns. Things if we shared on a first date, the person sitting across from us would get right up from the table and exit immediately.

No one is perfect. We are all flawed and have things about ourselves we are leery to share. In fear of being judged or misunderstood by someone we really like or want to know. Trust me, I get it. I picked up the terrible habit of smoking an occasional black and mild cigar after my breakup with AC to help deal with stress. After I kicked my black and mild habit, I found myself smoking cigarettes after work to compartmentalize the stress from work. That was my "secret behavior." I knew most people would be turned off by it and kept it tucked away, hidden. I would smoke in the same knitted hat, only outdoors, and in certain hoodies if it was cold outside. In my mind no one could detect a thing. But after a while, I let that habit go. It was too much that went into concealing the behavior: wearing certain clothing to smoke in, brushing my teeth immediately after, gum chewing galore, body spray, and hand sanitizer for the at-work organic American Spirit cigarette smoke session. Bottom line, we all got our secret stuff.

In life you also have to prepare yourself for people who will show up fully masked, camouflaging their authentic selves, like proclaiming they do not cheat when in fact they have never been monogamous in any relationship; promoting the word of God and all things Holy but quick to judge any and everyone for their shortcomings; claiming to be an amazing parent but talking about their child(ren)'s mother or father like a dog when they are impossible to co-parent with; exaggerating details about their life like being a nurse for example, when they may have started nursing school but did not finish. Eventually, the mask will slide or tilt to the side; the camouflage paint begins to smear, uncovering who they really are.

People may be embarrassed or insecure, so they play make believe for as long as possible in the beginning of starting something new. The goal is to reel you in, get you comfortable and emotionally invested. When they know you are in deep enough, they figure love or whatever you two have connected at this point (ex: children or a home) will more than likely make you stick around. It is wrong and selfish. However, when you discover who they are it is up to you to decide on where you go with this person. It is important to pay attention to people's actions in the beginning of a relationship. I cannot stress this enough. It will provide you a sneak peak of what your future will look like with this person. White lies in the beginning will likely lead to bigger lies later. If you do not want to take this on, do not allow this person to pass "go" and collect anymore of your time. Tell them "thanks for the date" and keep it pushin'! The age-old question that we all ask but can never answer about the person is: Can they change? Will they change? That is the risk we take sometimes on "love."

Journal Question:

How do you feel dating people with a rocky or questionable past but appear to have themselves together in the present? Is there such a thing as too much baggage? What can you deal with when dating someone new? Do you have baggage of your own that you feel is too much?

_____

_____

_____

_____

_____

_____

_____

_____

_____

_____

_____

_____

_____

_____

_____

_____

_____

_____

_____

_____

_____

"You can fool the whole world about who you truly are and
wear as many masks as you want. But at the end of the day
you lay in your own head, and you can't hide there."
—Danny Page 2.0

Chapter 22

Syllabi, Baby Rattles, and the Mirror on the Wall

Dominique

It can't be true! I was staring at the pregnancy test, waiting on that single blue line to pop up. I remember falling to my knees in tears as I saw the second blue line begin to appear. I thought, *My life is over! My parents are going to kill me, and I am not ready for this!*

I grabbed the stick, placed it in a piece of foil, and drove to Cleveland. I called Ishmael and told him we needed to talk face-to-face immediately. As he got in my car, I handed him the pregnancy test with tears in my eyes. He looked at me and said, "Why are you sad? I wanted you to have my child." I remember feeling some comfort but being more horrified by his response. I screamed, "We are nineteen, and I need to finish school!" He said, "Don't worry, we'll move in together and finish school."

Thankfully, my parents talked me into staying at home. I finished my bachelor's degree in four years, earning a Bachelor of Arts in social work. I went on to complete my master's degree from Case Western Reserve University by the age of twenty-three. I convinced myself I could have it all. A career and a family with my high school sweetheart, Ishmael.

Time after time, I took Ishmael back after countless incidents of cheating, children outside our relationship, arguments with "other" women, and more. I was broken, addicted, and clinging to an illusion of love. Once we had children, I was holding on to an idea of family. Yet somewhere on the inside, I knew I was confined to love's misery. We would break up to make up and jump into the toxic roller coaster ride we had both become accustomed to. Each relationship I had outside of Ishmael did NOT measure up if drama was not included.

Crushed by my choices, I did everything in my power to create a happy household. This was an attempt to sway him into becoming the father our children deserved and see my worth as a partner. However, my efforts didn't get me the picture-perfect outcome. In fact, I had another child with him at twenty-five. I started to realize I had the best parts of him in my beautiful daughter and son. Also, I learned love does NOT include disrespect and heartache. Though lessons were learned, it took a few more years of disappointment, frustration, and anger to sever ties for good and move on with my life. Once I opened myself up to the idea of change and moving forward, I began to focus on life, my dreams, and new beginnings.

Mirror Mirror on the Wall

Do you avoid mirrors and wear layers or colors that minimize your muffin top? If yes, you have met your newfound twin and sister in pain. But now, I have decided to live my life on purpose. I refuse to leave this earth with regrets from always living in the safe zone.

One of my favorite books is *The Dream Giver* by Bruce Wilkinson. The author tells a very simple yet powerful fable about a man named Ordinary, who knew he was meant for greater than the mundane of everyday life. Like Ordinary, I want to be great. I want to fulfill my dreams of helping those who have struggled with weight, self-esteem, and just life. My sister went up and down in her weight, but she never fully became the woman she fantasized about. I want to be the woman I have dreamed of my whole life. I want her to be proud and know I haven't forgotten the plan.

For many years I was trapped in a world of heartbreak and deception. I was so busy trying to avoid being labeled a statistic that I ran smack dead into it. I watched the man I had children with lie, cheat, and use me.

It was just 10 months after we had our first child that my world shattered. It was October 16, 2004—Sweetest Day, to be exact. I knew his behavior had changed, and I questioned that he might be cheating, but I didn't have proof. We were both juniors in college, and I refused to shack up. I knew I needed to finish college and have stability for my child, so I had moved back in with my parents. On this day I called his phone, and to my surprise a female answered. Confused and naive, I asked, "Well, where is Ishmael?" The female on the other end chuckled and said, "Oh, he's not here. I'll have him call you when he gets back home."

Back home? My mouth gaped open, and my heart was beating out of my chest. Paralyzed. *How could he do this to me, to us?* I hung up the phone and called his mother.

Side note: Women, why do we want to inflict pain on one another? No one wins in this scenario! Face it, he played the both of us.

His mother answered the phone. She consoled me, but it was clear I was the last to find out what everyone else already knew. When confronting Ishmael, he responded, "You chose to live with your parents, and I needed somewhere to live." At that moment, I realized the family I'd imagined was gone. I wish I could tell you I walked away, but I stayed hanging on to every lie he told me for the next three years.

Then the baby came. Finding out he had not only cheated but created a life with another woman was horrifying. The news broke my heart. Around the same time he welcomed his second child my health went haywire. I was rushed to the ER with a racing heart. The doctors hooked me up to oxygen and gave me a medication that stops your heart to reset it. I remember the fear of dying and the uncertainty. I spent the night in the hospital for observation, and doctors could not understand why my heart rate jumped up to 180 beats per minute when I stood up or switched positions. For the next year of my life, I spent every other night in the ER. The doctor diagnosed me with stress, depression, and panic attacks, but I knew it was more. At twenty-three, I weighed about 145 pounds, but I was miserable. For the first time in my life since childhood, I was an average weight, but my quality of life was poor. The doctors didn't know how to help, so they suggested I get a pacemaker. I was terrified! I was only twenty-three, in a graduate program at Case Western Reserve University.

I decided to take a chance on myself and God and do my own research. One day sitting in my parent's kitchen, I heard a highlight from a health specialist on television. I remember thinking, *Everything they're saying sounds like me.*

The next day I scheduled a doctor's appointment at University Hospital's neurology and cardiology departments. My cardiologist told me to increase my salt and fluids and exercise. With exercise and a tilt table test, it was evident I had POTS (Postural orthostatic tachycardia syndrome), an illness that attacks the sympathetic and parasympathetic nervous system. Finally, I had an answer, but life as I knew it had changed forever. My digestion, heart rate, blood pressure, and temperature were out of whack. The simplest things that most people do without thinking, such as walking or standing in line, were tasks for me.

To have a sense of stability and familiarity, I fell back into my old pattern. The moment Ishmael showed interest or apologized I went running to him. I had realized by now he was only a father when we were on good terms. He never took the time to bond with our daughter, but he had a connection with his new baby. I couldn't bring myself to look at the child he had with another woman. She represented the pain and betrayal I felt through years of lies and disappointments. I knew I needed to leave him, but I didn't know how.

Reflection:

I tricked myself into thinking I was different from her, his other woman. A lie many of us tell ourselves. I rode the roller coaster of destruction and self-sabotage for years to come. After every breakup, he had more children and baby mamas to show for it. I was gone, desperate, and in an abusive cycle that I had become addicted to. I prided myself on my detective skills—a female Columbo or Sherlock Holmes. I have looked through phone records and popped up at a few homes and had a few car chases, to say the least. It was not until my public display of rage and shame that I was pushed to my breaking point. I won't go into full detail, but let's just say I have a reputation of coming to blows at funerals. Yes, I know how it sounds, and trust I am a very different person now.

Many of us must transform our minds before we even begin to work on our outer appearance. Although I looked good on paper, I was a mess internally and began to hate the person I had become. I had painted the picture of being a strong and independent black woman, accomplishing everything I put my mind to, and I needed to become the type of woman and mother my children would be proud of. Sarah Jakes Roberts' book, *Lost and Found*, gave me a deeper understanding about the errors most of us make in love. Many of us are two broken and battered people entering relationships before doing the work to heal. Therefore, we add to each other's hurt in our own search for love and acceptance. I was forced to confront myself and see all my imperfections. I had to own my mistakes and take responsibility for my actions. We can blame our partner for hurting us, but we must first accept that part we played. Remember the old saying, a person can only do what we allow them to do. As hard as this statement is to accept, it is true.

Funny thing, people often say their partner completes them, but honestly, only God can fill those voids and broken spaces in our souls and our hearts. Our partner should simply complement us at best, not complete. Healing must take place within to truly accept or give genuine and unconditional love.

I have learned that we must forgive ourselves and reassure ourselves that we are worthy to receive love. As humans, we were created to be in relationships with others. I truly believe we were created to go through life together. No one is perfect, and we all hurt one another, both unintentionally and intentionally. The key is to discern the wolves disguised as sheep!

> "Life is tough, my darling, but so are you."
> —Stephanie Bennett-Henry

Today I forgive my children's father. I forgive him and accept him for who he is. I no longer want to argue or fight. I understand it is not my job to make him a man or father. I have removed the pressure of making our family work. I realize my sister was right all those years. Single mothers, know your children will be okay as long as you are. It takes a village to raise a child. The most important ingredient is love. As long as you provide love, affection, economic stability, and a strong support network for your children, I promise you they will thrive. Challenge yourself to be the person you imagined as a child. Having a child didn't count you out. A child is a gift that deserves to be nurtured.

Journal Question:

Have you felt betrayed by someone you dated? Can you identify with Dominique's struggle as a young or single mom? If yes, how?

_____

_____

_____

_____

_____

_____

_____

_____

_____

_____

_____

_____

_____

_____

_____

_____

_____

_____

_____

_____

"The saddest thing about betrayal is that it
never comes from your enemies"
—Unknown

Chapter 23

Running All Right

Ria

et us fast forward a bit. I accepted a new nursing position with the same company in Virginia that I was completely excited about! Kevin and I got engaged in Hawaii a year prior, and we agreed to start our lives in Virginia Beach. Immediately I thought what a great opportunity this would be for his kids, a new environment, better schools, finally working a routine schedule, I mean things were set! But in life things do not go as planned. Now there I was … post COVID in Virginia waiting for Kevin to show up. Oh, I know. Don't even get me started.

Per usual, I'd been going to Planet Fitness of course, but nothing was progressing with my weight loss as I hoped. Anticipating the Kevin and Ria wedding for 2021, I did not want to be as heavy as I was. I enlisted the assistance of a personal trainer, Jackson, in June of 2020. Kevin and I postponed our Virginia Beach wedding due to the Coronavirus aftermath: travel restrictions, business shutdowns, etc. My personal trainer, Jackson and I developed a natural bond over friendly conversations about work and relationships during our workouts. It was fall of 2020 during the last few sessions, I noticed that I would become teary-eyed when he'd ask how my week was. The truth was my week was f*****g terrible. My relationship with Kevin was fragile, and our arguments were constant. My fiancé and I were scheduled to see a new therapist who sounded promising. This weight of mine was at a standstill on the scale at 263-ish pounds.

My heaviest adult weight was 273 pounds around April of 2020. I started my journey with my trainer at 268 pounds. Although my measurements were moving in the right direction under Jackson's program, I was pissed! The scale was not moving as fast as I had hoped. Now don't get me wrong, we worked out two or three times a week, outside in the hot Virginia Beach sun and each session, he pushed me further. I think back to my first workout, and I applaud myself on where we ended. I was so out of breath on that first day—embarrassed even.

He would randomly record me during my session and text me the video later. I will admit, I was improving. It was also mortifying to watch myself and the person I saw, but damn it, I did NOT give up. I was angry, used plenty of swear words but I kept going. The person I saw was not beautiful, she looked miserable, unhappy, like she was tired of fighting. For years this woman had tried everything to lose weight: no carb diet, low carb diet, laxatives, apple cider vinegar, juicing, intermittent fasting, prescription weight loss pills, working out on my own, boot camps, personal training, hell I was exhausted. By the time we ended our workout relationship, I was stronger. My tolerance and weight resistance had gotten better, so that was growth, absolutely. Now, was I always 100 percent healthy with my food choices? No. But was I more mindful? Yes.

Unfortunately, I was mentally consumed by everything else at the time, like my love life, a wedding, the pandemic, and starting in a new clinic. Giving full attention to become a healthier version of myself was not there. Stress can do one of two things for your weight: add or subtract to it. My stress has always added pounds, plus some. As I got older, the number on the weighted stress scale jumped higher and higher adding more pressure on myself to change it.

During our last training session at Planet Fitness, I showed up with the worst, nonchalant, funky Cancerian attitude. Jackson could tell, and that night he was over my b******t. We were on the treadmill, mid-conversation, about the workout ahead that evening and I blurted out, "I'm just going to get weight loss surgery anyway. That's what I'm going to do." Jackson asked why. I said something along the lines of, "The scale isn't moving, and I'm tired of putting in this work with no results. The scale says I'm still fat, and I'm wasting money." My trainer and I went back and forth for a minute or so like boyfriend and girlfriend. Then, he left me right there in Planet Fitness. I mean … *walked … right … out.* Me being me, I yelled out, "Bye!" in the most stank way, eyes rolling and all, and continued my workout for the evening.

When I got into my car, I was surprised to settle into my little SUV and see a three-minute voicemail from Jackson that was actually quite supportive. I remember texting him back as I pulled into my parking to apologize. I felt bad about our public disagreement but relieved about my decision to pursue what I felt was best for my health. Our personal training relationship door closed that day; it was the last time I paid anyone to train and get me together too.

After Jackson, I resumed my own gym schedule at Planet Fitness while researching options for bariatric surgery in my area. I attended an in-person session and committed myself to a lengthy process of a lifestyle change with Chesapeake Regional Medical Center. For years, my mother tried talking me into weight loss surgery, the sleeve gastrectomy. She went through it herself, becoming very successful in maintaining her more slender frame, obsessing over her OrangeTheory Fitness classes. When I started my government job in 2013, I attempted a bariatric surgery program with St. Vincent Hospital in Cleveland, Ohio. I was four months in, prepared to get my pre-op lab work, then flaked. I used the excuse "Well, I'm sure I will have kids in the future, so why do this surgery now …, blah blah blah …"

See how that turned out? I'm in my very late thirties with no children and multiple fibroids that need to be removed. Besides, if I had done it then, I am not sure how committed I would have been to the aftercare process. The changes in lifestyle are drastic to maintain the weight loss, especially within the first year. In 2013, I was younger, still going out, and making reckless decisions with my waistline as well as my heart. It didn't seem like that type of commitment was going to make the cut.

Reflection:

Looking back on my attitude toward Jackson, I was a major b***h. Seriously. He was showing up to help me become a better version of myself. I was showing up rude as f**k like everything I felt going wrong in my life was his doing. I've apologized numerous times to him up to this day. We've since talked about it, and he did not train anyone for a while after our big blowout. This brings me to a great point: you see how our actions affect the people in our lives? Now, don't get it confused. Jackson is doing well and has ventured into other avenues, bringing him joy in other ways. But it is bothersome to know my piss-poor attitude had that great of an impact on him when that was never my intention. Jackson, I am not that same person anymore, miserable in her own skin. I'm shedding those old layers every day. I appreciate everything you taught me during our time together. Even though you had me working out in the hot blazing sun ... in the grass with garden snakes unbeknownst to me.

It is our responsibility to check our baggage at the door when we enter spaces with other people. At home, work, events, the gym, wherever. Unless you are meeting up to discuss your life and what's going on in it, check yourself. Our dirty or wrinkled laundry does not need to spill into the laps of other people without their permission. We have to remind ourselves there is a time and place for everything. When we are engaging in activities that are intended to empower, restore, or improve ourselves, leave the negative energy at the damn door. It's unfair to the people attempting to share the positive aura around you, and it's unfair to the person who is trying to better themselves ... *You*. We are quick to hold other people accountable for their actions, but there comes a few times when we need to take a look in the mirror and do the exact same. Be the type of person toward others that you want them to be toward you—decent, respectful.

When you have overstepped boundaries, and the person you may have offended has told you, apologize. Why? Because something you said or did hurt their feelings, made them feel some type of way. When you are going through something personal (minor or major) figure out the best way to deal with your emotions to avoid misdirecting your anger on the wrong people. Journaling, screaming into a pillow every morning, prayer, punching the couch pillow, meditation, or therapy. Anything that can relieve the stress you are dealing with to avoid it becoming public. It is never easy to walk around with the weight of the world on your shoulders. Eventually, you will hit a breaking point from the smallest thing like a cashier at Chick-fil-A forgetting to say, "Have a great day." The next thing you know someone is recording your argument at the drive-thru window for Tik Tok while you're screaming, "F**k you, little Chick-fil-A b***h. I hope your little boyfriend is talking to a bunch of hoes too. Now give me my extra Polynesian sauce with my nuggets." It does not need to go there. It is hard while we are going through personal matters, multiple things at once and we want to know "why is this happening?"

God will test us for reasons we will never understand, but the pain has purpose. We do not understand it in the midst of the storm but believe me, He is testing you.

Journal Question:

Have you ever taken your anger out on a person attempting to help you make a positive change? Did you attempt to apologize and was it accepted?

_____

_____

_____

_____

_____

_____

_____

_____

_____

_____

_____

_____

_____

_____

_____

_____

_____

_____

_____

_____

_____

_____

_____

"Make peace with your broken pieces."
—RH Sin

Chapter 24

The Girl is Mine

Dominique

I was in my mid-twenties and expecting my second child. I had a new sense of clarity and a fresh outlook on life. It's funny how traumatic life events bring us face-to-face with our mortality and the need to make necessary life changes. Desperate and ashamed, I went against my better judgment and chose to move in with Ishmael. I felt I owed it to our four-year-old daughter to give her a real family. I tricked myself into thinking he would be faithful if we lived together. However, I felt trapped and confused. We rented a small two-bedroom apartment and ran up my Value City Furniture credit card to furnish it. If you're wondering if he continued to cheat during my pregnancy, the answer is yes.

I began working at a local mental health agency with children and adolescents. I was beginning to blossom professionally, and I was maintaining my weight loss and small frame during my pregnancy. My POTS appeared to be in remission, and I felt like myself again. However, I chose to hide my pregnancy from family and friends until I couldn't hide it anymore.

Stressed with my new living arrangements, secret pregnancy, and make-up-to-break-up drama, I was at my wit's end. It was my birthday. I was seven months pregnant, dressed, and ready for work. I walked out to the parking lot and noticed both of my back tires were flat. Confused, thinking my eyes were playing tricks on me, I walked closer to my vehicle to get a better look. Immediately, I noticed both of my back tires were slashed.

I ran back into the house and woke Ishmael. He looked at me dazed and confused and told me to calm down. I asked him who would slash my tires. He said, "I told you to stop sleeping with married men." At that moment, I lost it and charged at him. He restrained me and assured me that he had nothing to do with the mishap I was facing. Holding back tears, I called my parents and asked for help. My mother calmly told me to come over and get her Sears card to purchase two new tires. Ishmael drove me to Sears in his brand-new Dodge Charger (which was in my name) to buy my tires. He never admitted any fault or apologized for ruining my birthday.

I was tired and fed up with his actions. Although I didn't have any proof, I knew it was a scorned woman who slashed my tires. That day, I made up my mind and moved back in with my parents. You see, I had never fully committed to living with Ishmael. In arguments, he would often mention how I never moved all my belongings in. I believe deep down I knew living together was a bad idea. But I wanted to give our four-year-old daughter and new addition a stable home, so I handed him my set of keys and came to terms with the thought of raising my children alone.

At that moment, I understood my children deserved a mother who chose them and not a dysfunctional relationship. For so long, I was focused on my relationship with Ishmael and failed to recognize the impact our decisions had on our children. I reminisced on the countless arguments and tears I shed in front of our children. The love I had for my children superseded my dependency and love for their father. I wanted more. To experience the love of a man who wanted me and my children. Someone who was willing to build a life with me, in a monogamous relationship.

After the birth of our son, I was ready for something new. I received a Facebook message from Derrick, my high school crush. We had first met at the age of sixteen while he was working at a local pizzeria. He was tall, dark, handsome, and charming. Our birthdays were two days apart, and we clicked. I always liked Derrick, but he was notorious for playing mind games during our adolescence, so I was cautious when he first reached out. I waited until Thanksgiving to give him a call. He told me he had gone to the military and matured a great deal since we were children. I was intrigued and decided to see where this old flame could take me. Derrick showed interest in me as an overweight teen, and I was hoping he would find interest in the smaller frame I had worked so hard to maintain. I appreciated Derrick's confidence and the way he made me feel when we were together. He reassured me of his interest, however, I could not shake the feeling that he was hiding something.

We dated, and he often told me about the future he hoped to have with me. Everything seemed to be going well until I received a call from Sophia. I was in a continuing education class for my social work license when my phone rang. I remember the phone number was blocked, and I decided to answer. The person on the other end began to ask me if I knew someone named Derrick. I thought, *Here we go again!* Taking a deep breath, I answered yes. I then asked the person their name and why they called me. The person said, "My name is Sophia, and Derrick is in the shower. I just wanted to know who you are." She went on to say, "Your name is listed as 'Mine' in his phone."

In shock, I asked Sophia, "Who are you, Derrick?"

Crying, she answered, "I don't know. I am whoever he wants me to be."

Reflection:

Have you ever asked yourself why you continue to attract or date the same person? Different name, but the same person. I have asked myself this question more times than I would like to admit. I left my children's father to enter a courtship with a man who exhibited the same behaviors and possessed some of the same characteristics. I fell in love with Derrick, but I thought I was undeserving of real love due to the trauma I experienced in my relationship with Ishamel.

Sophia and I were both victims of his lies and deception. Many of us start relationships without ending the one we are currently in. As cliché as it may sound, honesty is key in love. No one deserves to be treated like a pawn in a game of chess. Years later, Derrick apologized, allowing us to become friends—a friendship that was never pure or appeared genuine.

Due to my previous interest in Derrick and poor self-image, I allowed him to use me. Yet, looking back I see how my relationship with him was just as damaging as my relationship with Ishmael. I allowed both men to use me for what they could acquire from our relationship, whether it was emotional or financial support. Neither party respected me or took accountability for their actions if they hurt or disappointed me. I thought I was safe in the friend zone, but Derrick used this title to his advantage. He would go out of his way to remind me of our friend status when it was convenient. Yet, in private often in a drunken stupor, he would profess his love. I found myself confused and waiting for him to choose me. You see, this is the cycle I was stuck in. I was hanging in the background waiting for men (who were in fact abusing me emotionally) to finally see and love me. But they never did.

Regardless of my genuine love for him, he failed to reciprocate the loyalty or love I displayed. I was his companion when he was lonely and dropped whenever he was entertaining the woman of the month. He affectionately referred to me as his "DB" to all his friends and family. I looked forward to our wakeup phone calls and nightly chats. Our friendship became an important piece of my identity and daily routine. Willingly, I accepted his secret devotion to me, although he rejected me publicly. I remember Christmas was approaching, and we had not planned on exchanging gifts, however, he let it slip that he bought me a gift. I was shocked that he thought of me and felt special. In a rush to show my appreciation, I went to Ulta and bought Gucci Guilty, a cologne I heard him reference in conversation.

Fast forward to Christmas Day, I was excited to exchange gifts. I remember opening the door to an empty-handed Derrick; I was shocked! He grabbed me around my waist and began to hug me and said, "I didn't get you anything, but I will make it up to you, I promise!" Trying not to show my disappointment, I said okay and walked him out. A few hours later he called me while in the car with one of his friends. I heard his friend on the other end saying, "You got a good girl, Derrick!" Derrick quickly corrected him and said, "This is my homie, my dogg, not my girl!" Now, I didn't expect him to say we were more than friends, but I was embarrassed and felt the underlying rejection of his words. Later in the week, Derrick told me about the bracelets he bought a new love interest for Christmas. Livid, I ended our conversation abruptly. Aware that he had upset me, he called back and told me he was giving me a month's worth of eyebrow threading services as my Christmas gift. Less than pleased, I accepted his gift because I felt he owed me. I knew I had to emotionally detach from him. Our relationship was draining and wasn't going anywhere.

Ladies, we have to stop waiting in the background for our love interest to notice us. I was blinded by my love for Derrick. Like Ishmael, he made promises that he never fulfilled. If you find yourself befriending someone who is emotionally unavailable, move on if you are in search of marriage or a committed relationship.

Although Derrick and I were not involved sexually, I provided him with the emotional benefits of a relationship without the title. Now don't get me wrong, he provided me with companionship as well. Yet, I wanted more, and he was not ready or willing to meet my needs. Our interaction forced me to question myself. He told me I was beautiful, but his actions made me feel he was ashamed to be with me. What was wrong with me? Why didn't he want me? I was tormenting myself by staying stuck in a friendship that was one-sided. Do not wait on other people to determine your fate!

Now looking back, maybe he was just flirtatious, and I was misreading our interactions. We remain cordial, but our friendship has changed drastically. I learned to accept Derrick for who he was. So often we try to change people or have unrealistic expectations for people based on our wants and desires. I accepted that there may have been past hurt or insecurities that made Derrick the way he was, or maybe he truly just wanted to be my friend, in which I had to check my ego. I will forever have a genuine love for Derrick due to the advice and time we shared. It's clear we were not each other's match and that's okay.

This experience taught me to avoid dating people who send mixed messages. I urge you to be confident in what you have to offer in a relationship and don't waiver or change your mind because of their double-mindedness. A man who wants you to know you are just friends has no intention of being your man, trust me! Make yourself emotionally available to someone who is sure of what they want and is interested in you and only you. I found that distancing myself from Derrick helped me move forward. I stopped making myself accessible to him at all times of the day and night and began to date. If you find yourself in a similar situation and are ready for real love, try declining phone calls and invitations to hang out with the one who has put you in the friend zone. This allows you to create space in your life to date again. Tell yourself that you deserve more!

Journal Question:

Have you found yourself in a friendship or dating someone who is emotionally unavailable? If yes, how has this affected your self-esteem and outlook on love?

_____

_____

_____

_____

_____

_____

_____

_____

_____

_____

_____

_____

_____

_____

_____

_____

_____

_____

_____

_____

_____

_____

_____

_____

"Love is not what you say. Love is what you do."
—Unknown

Chapter 25

If the Sleeve Fits

———

Ria

Halfway into 2021, I was scheduling my appointments with the bar-iatric surgeon, Dr. Hui, and his team one by one. The discussion on which procedure to plan for (gastric sleeve versus gastric bypass), completing labs/chest x-ray, liver ultrasound, esophagogastroduodenoscopy (EGD), a psychiatry appointment, participating in nutrition appointments over a four-month period.

The nutrition appointments were the most difficult. My surgeon required me to lose five to ten pounds on my own, which was easy enough. But the nutritionist, Lori, always wanted to talk and ask me how my week was going. Very normal line of questioning anyone would ask, but at the time it was always a sore subject because it was never going well. Such a trigger for me. I would think, *Damn, why can't I just get on the scale, total up these little pounds and head back to work?* My emotions were always everywhere. Praying my menstrual cycle weight wouldn't affect my weigh-in requirement for Dr. Hui or hoping her "How's it going" question would not break me down into tears. My relationship with Kevin had been rocky for some time; he was constantly traveling with his new career of entrepreneurship, and I was living in Virginia alone. This will be explained later.

Over time, I learned the meaning behind mind over matter. Every day I was learning to wake up with the intention to complete small goals. For example, prepping work lunches on Sundays, or cooking dinner after work versus DoorDashing. I started to apply the information from my appointments, such as not drinking with meals thirty minutes before and after, measuring meal portions, and reading the nutrition labels (actually eating the one-serving size).

I could not stand the nutritionist Lori (she was actually a nice lady). She was slender with perfect shoulder-length hair and her engagement ring rested beautifully on her finger. I would often think about my generic responses to her question: "It's going okay, it could be worse," or "Well, it's all right." We would sit there going over what to expect in the upcoming months, food choices, how to use food, and vitamin tracking apps, etc. The entire time I would stare at her engagement ring and wonder what type of relationship issues she had at home, if any. Does her husband think she's pretty? What does she really eat at home? Is she happy? Me? Well, I'm here planning one of the biggest events of my life, and my fiancé is well, you know, in Cleveland or Atlanta or wherever. All I knew was he was not where he was supposed to be: settled in Virginia with me.

By April 2021, I completed my pre-surgical requirements. I recall my last nutritionist appointment sobbing with joy in her office. I hate to admit it, but in the height of an emotional moment I sometimes cry just like that (finger snap).

"Well, Ria, I'm happy to inform you that you've been approved for surgery." It was the best news I'd heard in a long time. She didn't realize what it meant for me. (I know she also probably hears this a few times a week from other patients). I rattled off all the activities I couldn't wait to try for the first time, like horseback riding and returning to Cedar Point for some roller coaster rides. In the midst of my excitement, I may have shared with her a future Gucci bikini purchase. She saw how important the moment was for me, and she smiled.

Once a storm hits and everything settles, there's a calmness in the air, earthly renewal. It was May 2021, almost that time when fellow Cancerians unite and prepare for birthday trips, summer holiday celebrations, and basking in the sun (can y'all feel it?).

My relationship with Kevin was feeling more like an atomic bomb ready to explode at any minute. Love was wearing me down. Officially entering a space where I needed individual therapy, aside from couples therapy. Now that is deep. It became clear the relationship I was in and out of, where I once felt confident, left me unsure of myself. I needed professional help and quickly. In May of 2021, Kevin decided after one argument surrounding his trip to Virginia that we needed to take a break from each other, but the engagement was still on. What kind of s**t is that?

After speaking with my personal therapist, Coach K, and doing some soul sailing, I realized I would be good no matter what I would decide for myself. I've gone through so much with men (from the past and Kevin in the present). Reality was settling into my heart: what love is and is NOT. Like, if it ain't giving what it's supposed to, I gotta head out 🏃. Besides reclaiming my self-worth, I was looking forward to snatched summer seasons in my future. Hopefully, by the time you read this, I will be half-naked, tanning poolside in an overpriced luxury brand swimsuit with matching slides "just because".

Reflection:

Sounds like simple steps to follow. Read the food labels, measure your food, workout, and do right. Wrong. Wrong, and wrong if you are not in the proper mental state to practice what you are learning. I will say this, when you are fed the hell up and reach your breaking point, you just do it. You wake up and realize, "Self, this is what I want, and we just gotta do what we gotta do." I was done with inconsistent dieting, improper eating, and working out without continued success for maintaining weight loss. I was tired of limiting my shopping to the online plus-size filters at Gap, Old Navy, and Fashionova. This woman got sick of wearing modest two-piece bathing suits and no longer fitting comfortably into a size 38C bra from Victoria's Secret. Hear me out: "Just Do It." Stop slacking on yourself coming up with excuses holding yourself back from the next level of YOU. It is easy to get comfortable where you are and turn a blind eye to what the outcome could be. Make the adjustments already! It is unfamiliar in the beginning. Like riding a bike with no training wheels, it takes getting used to, but it will be worth it.

I missed riding roller coasters, mentally spent by worrying if certain rides had sturdy cords and belt straps that safely secured heavier people or fit across my lap. I was tired of sitting out on the sidelines lying to people, "I'm afraid of heights," when the truth was, I didn't feel comfortable. Hell, I wanna go horseback riding into the sunset, but I don't want to throw Black Beauty's back out! There was a whole world out there for me to explore, and year after year, it was passing me by. I had allowed the numbers on the scale to rip away life and fashion moments from me. Enough was enough.

With that being said, the happiest days of some people's lives are life milestones like graduations, marriage, buying a home, or giving birth. Hearing my surgery approval had officially become one of mine. Do not get me wrong, I've had other life accomplishments to celebrate, but this was an official life-changing chapter to Ria G. This next chapter would be filled with trying new things without feeling insecure, true unfiltered shopping, and actually living life. Sure, there would be hiccups along the way, but the positives would outweigh the negatives.

Life is too short to be confined in a cage of self-doubt and hesitancy, hiding behind fake smiles and "perfect" angles for the rest of your life. Stop being the master at pretending to be happy and take any opportunity to just *be* happy. Keep your needs a priority and understand happiness will not be found in anyone other than yourself. Explore new hobbies, revisit an old skill, or invest in self-care like a monthly massage. To the people pleasers out there, this one is especially for you: STOP. It is going to be a nasty habit to break, and you will feel guilty too, but stop trying to make everyone's else's day go as smooth as ice. Take a stance on this, ten toes down and start telling people "No." Get comfortable with the idea you are no longer people pleasing, staged for an audience of people who don't matter, angled and sucked in for people who couldn't care less. The people who want to see you win will be there at your worst or best, carrying you along the way to the finish line.

Journal Question:

What attempts have you made to engage in a healthy lifestyle change? Were you successful? If so, what was helpful? If not, can you identify what could have been the cause?

_____

_____

_____

_____

_____

_____

_____

_____

_____

_____

_____

_____

_____

_____

_____

_____

_____

_____

_____

_____

_____

"You can't go back and change the beginning, but you can start where you are and change the ending."
—C.S. Lewis

Chapter 26

The Weight Gain...
If I Lived Down South

Dominique

A fter losing weight in college, I maintained my weight loss until the age of 27. You know, I am still unsure what changed during this period in my life. The weight came back slowly. First 10, then 20 pounds, and before I knew it, I had gained 50 pounds. I was devastated, to say the least. I was a single mother of two, working as a grief counselor. Sure, I had emotional baggage like the next woman. But, as I began to see the numbers go up on the scale, I started to panic. I remember the fear creeping up in my chest. The fear of being *"fat."* Fearful of not being seen as beautiful to myself and others. The fear of my childhood experiences and suffering through the same emotions as an adult.

I tried fad diets, meal plans, boot camps, and more. It seemed no matter what I did, though, the pounds kept coming, and so did feelings of depression. Those old feelings of inadequacy and negative self-talk started to resurface. I reverted to the little girl who felt judged and stifled by her weight. All those memories came rushing in like a flash flood, no consideration, no care, nothing.

Feeling like a failure, I often thought, *How did I let myself go again?* I was determined to shed the extra weight I gained. I dreaded seeing 180 pounds on the scale. Immediately, I began to search for exercise equipment online to build myself a home gym. I found a treadmill for $700 dollars on Sears.com and couldn't wait to get started. Once I placed it in my basement, I promised myself I would workout three to four times per week. After a couple of weeks, I found myself becoming discouraged as the numbers of the scale didn't budge. I just knew I needed to execute plan B, Jenny Craig. I scheduled an appointment and was ready to meet with my fitness coach. She encouraged me to set short-term goals and find the link between my emotional triggers that may cause me to overeat. I realize now that I was not in the proper mindset to identify my triggers that led to me overindulge in kettle-style chips or other snacks. I just wanted to feel good about myself and see the pounds melt away. Afterward, I found that eating packaged food was even harder than being mindful of my emotions. I was bored. Although many of the meals were tasty, I was not determined to continue the program. So I quit. I was back at square one with no idea what I was going to do. Instead of looking within, I turned to another relationship to fix me. Big mistake!

If I lived Down South

I was approaching 30, and I began dating a guy named Cedric, whom I met after my first daughter was born. We worked as AmeriCorps volunteers and had what seemed to be an instant connection. I remember thinking he had a slight arrogance that intrigued me. He was a fan-favorite among the women we worked with. To be honest, I think I sought him out because I saw him as a conquest. We flirted and occasionally hung out and always had great conversations, both valuing education and family, but he never admitted to having any interest in me. I was not fully over my children's father and unsure of Cedric's intentions, and we drifted apart.

Over the years, we found our way back to each other. I was ready for a new experience, and 30 was knocking at the door. I thought, why not? What do I have to lose? Now, he wasn't someone I was physically attracted to, but our mental and emotional connections outweighed the physical, or so I thought. He was into physical fitness and loved training people to reach their fitness goals.

Problems in our relationship started when he made me feel judged and uncomfortable in my skin. By this point in life, I was done allowing anyone to make me feel bad about myself. Why would I? I was educated, career-oriented, and a homeowner before 29. I knew I was a catch! He loved complimenting me but also made sure to catapult subtle shade from time to time. He judged me by comparing me to his mother. Suggesting I was weak for staying with my children's father for so long. I struggled with feeling the need to defend myself against the man who told me he hoped to have a future with me.

Prime example: It was New Year's Eve, and I was wearing a tunic sweater, skinny jeans, and thigh-high leather boots. Beyond ready for our double date to bring in the new year. As I walked through the door, he grinned and said, "Butler, see they would be all over you if you lived down south," referencing how Southern men love their women on the thicker side. I looked at him and said, "What does that mean?" His response: "Oh, you know I'm just joking ..."

From that moment on, I remember thinking, *Here goes another person who has a problem with my weight.* Due to his ignorant comment and other comments to follow, let's just say the relationship didn't last.

Reflection:

Let's be very honest: The battle of losing and gaining weight is exhausting! I can't count the number of times I have wished I could snap my fingers, lose weight, and lay on the beach in a two-piece bikini. I hate the demands society places on women and the inner turmoil women go through to meet those demands. Life can be unfair.

I know some people will say get over it ... weight is superficial or it's truly not that hard to lose weight. I have tried personal training and dieting. I have lost and I have gained. It's not about laziness for me. So my advice is not to get discouraged by the naysayers but to do what is best for you—whether that is weight-loss surgery, exercise, diet, or nothing at all. Find happiness in you! Try not to find happiness in the man or woman you are dating. You must do the work to heal first. Take the time out to get to know you. A famous quote by Alicia Ramos, says "A woman who realizes her worth, is a dangerous woman." When we recognize our worth, we no longer allow the words of others to define us. We no longer allow those around us to change who we are or who we want to become.

You should not have to prove your beauty or worth to anyone! Never settle. Allow better to find you. It's funny. I followed everyone's advice instead of listening to that inner voice we all have inside. So many of my friends said, "You will learn to love him," or "He is a good man. You deserve to be treated right." Yes, they were right. I *do* deserve to be treated right, but forcing yourself to fall in love will lead to nothing but disaster in the end. I appreciate Cedric showing me how a man should build a partnership with a woman and respect her children if he desires to be in a long-term relationship with a single mother. Cedric never attempted to sleep over my house or lay in the bed with me while my children were at home. Which made me respect him.

The truth is he was a good man; he just wasn't right for me. For so long I thought I was shallow and was looking for all the wrong attributes in a mate. Now I see that attraction is huge! Do you hear me? Huge!

Yes, I learned that love goes way beyond a physical or sexual attraction, but one should exist. Cedric and I had chemistry in terms of our communication, but we had different values. I had to be honest with myself and let him go. I could have married him, but I never would have accepted him or truly been happy. Both he and I deserved better.

To Cedric, I apologize for hurting you and hope you found true love. But you didn't love me. You were in love with an idea of who you wanted me to be. You never loved me for me and attempted to change me to fit your picture of your ideal woman. As I tried to change you as well, which wasn't fair to either of us.

Journal Question:

Have you felt judged in your relationship before? Have you found yourself dating someone you are not attracted to? If yes, why?

_____

_____

_____

_____

_____

_____

_____

_____

_____

_____

_____

_____

_____

_____

_____

_____

_____

_____

_____

_____

_____

_____

"I walked away because you were too busy finding
faults in me while I was busy overlooking yours."
—Unknown

Chapter 27

The BIG Bang

Ria

Surgery dates are typically given weeks in advance to give you time to plan for work and people to have on standby for support. Excited to have time off from work, I was looking forward to much needed rest and relaxation from the day-to-day nurse grind. I've never experienced extended time away from work, and my relationship had been pushing me over the edge emotionally.

I left work early one afternoon after a back-and-forth text conversation with my "?" (I'm not sure what he was that day: fiancé, boyfriend, friend, enemy ...). There was a Titanic full of tears behind my eyes, ready to capsize at any moment. I refused to sit there in front of my computer and pretend to be okay. Swallowing my pride, I politely excused myself via Microsoft Teams to my nurse manager. Thank God Nurse E was cool, and I had plenty of comp time to use. I remember calling Dominique in tears like someone had just died. She could barely understand me, and I felt foolish. But she understood why without me saying a word.

In the text conversation, he told me he needed to work on being a better man, told me I did not bring him peace, and this is why he needed a break from our relationship. Yes, the relationship that we are engaged in, that's right.

With the wedding in a complete gray area, my surgery date became set in stone, July 7, 2021. Kevin and I were still on speaking terms. He planned to spend a week or two with me during recovery. I looked forward to us spending time together and thought this would help fix our problems. We'd been living apart for a year and a half now and had more downs than ups at this point.

If you recall, the original plan was for us to relocate to Virginia in November 2019, have our beach wedding in June 2020, and live happily. I moved to Virginia Beach first in November 2019. The same night after we settled in, Kevin said, "Hey, I won't be here until January 2020 (not what we discussed). As time went by (months into 2020), so did Kevin's relocation date to Virginia. His belongings and important documents made it to our townhouse and storage unit, however, Kevin did not. By fall of 2020, I knew he had no intentions on relocating to Virginia. I figured moving back to Ohio was my next move to show my support for him and his new endeavors.

Kevin never voiced an issue with my weight. When I met him, I was probably in the high 230s and gained about 30 pounds during our six-year relationship, with weight loss back and forth in between. After making the decision to have bariatric surgery, he said, "Okay, if that's what you wanna do." But the tone was different. It was not one of excitement but more like, "Oh, okay, do you, buddy." During the months of my preparation, he rarely, if at all, asked about my appointments or seemed interested when I talked about them. His attitude came off as if he did NOT care. My friends and family were my cheer squad, excited for me taking this huge leap into health transformation. But the one person whose support I needed the most? ... Nah.

The last "Big Girl" birthday trip before my health and wellness journey June 2021 was unforgettable. I was looking forward to spending it with Kevin in Miami; we usually have fun on vacation. Sun tanning, the beach, day drinking, good food, and bae to myself for a few days. I mean, what could go wrong? Oh, well ... everything. I mean, everything from the partly cloudy yet sunny Floridian skies was off. Simply weird and not right. From sitting separately on the plane to Miami and the awkward conversations during breakfast and dinner the entire trip. There is nothing worse than being on a trip with someone you love and still feel so far away from them. I would've found more comfort in a white padded room.

On my actual birthday, I felt like a complete idiot. I was sitting poolside, initially drinking alone, until I linked up with some pretty, thick bodied sisters from Houston, Texas. Welp, here I am oiled up, hair in a messy bun with black Marc Jacobs shades resting on top, and in my best American Eagle two-piece swimsuit. Kevin was in the middle of taking an online course monopolizing his entire time on our trip. Well, minus the two hours or so he spent at the pool one day out of the three-day weekend. A cringe-worthy moment with complimentary drinks, the sun kissing my back because it definitely was not Kevin. Everything was a vibe except for us. He did an amazing job making me feel unwanted during this trip: barely looking in my direction, touching or talking to me when he did decide to bless me with his presence.

Do you know how simple I felt when the sisters from Houston asked, "Are you here by yourself?" during one of many moments by the pool. It wasn't just the sisters either; it was everyone I had a conversation with that day: "Awww, it's your birthday! Wait, are you here by yourself?" Baby, never again will I do that to myself on a trip with any damn one.

Two days before surgery, July 5, 2021, Kevin asked if I really wanted him at the hospital. Once he posed that question, I knew he was not staying the entire week, let alone two. My summer so far had been conversations with him telling me: "I think it's best I take a break from this relationship so I can become a better man," and "You don't bring me peace when I come home." It would be difficult to have a sense of peace if one is living a double life. It was later revealed he had become "close" with a female business partner behind my back. Someone he introduced to me about four years prior. Surely, keeping all the lies straight can become tiresome if you think about it. Telling me one thing and your "business partner" another. My favorite quote that kept me strapped into the ride of hell and heartbreak: "We just need to get back on track."

Kevin's flight was delayed due to weather the day of my surgery, so it was another moment of too little too late. He barely made it after I was cut open and pushed into the hospital room for the night. My mother was not happy and did not plan for this unexpected change of plans. Not only was he late, but he was not even staying? This was another slash mark in her notepad against him.

I remember Kevin being extremely attentive in those twelve hours during my hospitalization. It was the most genuine care and concern he'd expressed in months; this was the person I missed. But when I was discharged home the next day, he was back in Cleveland not even 24-hours later. No worries on my end, best friend TJ showed up within the next 48-hours with his Louis Vuitton duffle bag over his shoulder. TJ couldn't believe how quickly old boy purchased his flight back home but was not surprised. The first few days in my post-op recovery, Kevin was not really checking in on me, asking how I felt or how I was doing—just pure not-giving-a-f**k behavior. I thought, *This man really doesn't give a damn …*

During TJ's visit, the roller coaster from hell beginning in May extended the ride time when an unknown IG message found its way into my Instagram direct messages (DM). It was the kind of message everyone dreads about their significant other. The DM came from an unknown female that went along these lines, "I'm not trying to break up a happy home … I know you're his fiancée … he was at an event holding hands with this female …" It is the moment you ask yourself, "Should I check this shit out?" In the back of your mind, your intuition has been nudging you for months, so you do what most women would do in my position: hit reply. "Hey, sis, what's up?" To clarify, this unknown woman reached out to me a second time shortly after, attempting to offer me words of encouragement like, "Yeah, women need to stick together. I don't like to see people getting done wrong." For her not to know me, she sure had my back, or did she? It doesn't matter, the information allowed me to trade in those rose-colored Ray Bans for the transparent Gucci eyewear I needed.

My rest and recovery from work turned into a full-blown investigation while I adapted to my new life after bariatric surgery. The lifestyle changes required mental and emotional commitment for the best outcome: rigid vitamin schedule, new volume fluid intake, barely tolerating soft foods, and learning how to dodge severe constipation. I refused to let episodes of my own "Livin La Vida Loca" throw me off course. The gym and I reconnected much sooner than allowed, but it saved me. Every morning I got up and drove straight to Planet Fitness, walking the treadmill for about thirty minutes or so. As weeks went by, I increased my incline and reintroduced weights into my mix. Once the pool opened for the day, I would lay out for a few hours, tan, indulge on sugar-free popsicles, and read. That was my morning and mid-day routine the rest of summer.

I was about 30 pounds lighter and ready to return to work. Despite how I felt emotionally, people kept telling me about the glow I possessed. I credit it to my lazy poolside afternoons soaking up natural vitamin D, attempting to decompress. It was difficult to hide the internal house fire I was surviving, unless you were my inner circle then you knew about the blaze. It was a traumatic experience I wouldn't wish on anyone. No matter how many firefighters showed up to extinguish the fire with me, it seemingly grew bigger week after week. New information to process was nonstop: Kevin's "business partner" started posting pictures and videos of them together on dinner dates, at the mall (as he attempted to run out of one video trying not to be recorded), and subliminal IG posts that seemed directed toward me for months.

One weekend a few weeks after surgery, I even came home and found his truck parked in an Extended Stay hotel parking lot. This was the following morning after he ignored my calls and text. The same person who complained "I never come to Cleveland to visit." Oddly enough, I came home, and he ghosted me after the truth began to unfold … huh. His truck was parked right next to his business partner's vehicle at seven in the morning. Coincidence?

I am forever indebted to the two women who answered their phones that morning. Once I woke up I knew something wasn't right. My female intuition said, "B**h, look at those pictures again …" Strategically, I matched up headboards from pictures on Expedia, doing a search for Cleveland area hotels. Immediately, I threw my clothes on from the night before and darted out the house. An intense rage rushed through my veins when I pulled into that dusty ass hotel parking lot. My friends pleaded over the phone, "Ria, please don't do it. They have cameras in those parking lots. He isn't worth going to jail over." There was nothing but a f******g river streaming down my face, looking a mess. I didn't leave without any proof because I wanted to know what story Kevin would provide. There was always an explanation. After I pulled my shit together, I sent him a text with the picture of both vehicles. He had the audacity to tell me he let his "other" business partner use his truck for a business meeting that morning at this hotel. Okay, Kevin …

My efforts were pushed to the max toward becoming a better me on the outside. Emotionally, I reached my limit on love with Kevin. That time allowed me to evaluate everything that occurred pre and post-surgery between us. It was time to walk away. Multiple events occurring over the last few months were not his first acts of reasonable doubt in our relationship. There was an episode of infidelity early on, when I thought our relationship was "perfect." He decided to have sex with an ex-girlfriend and thought they had twins on the way. Of course he was not forthcoming about this. Again, my intuition at the time led me to this information. We separated for months and no children came from his act of indiscretion. During our break, he went out of his way to "prove" his love for me. Gifts, tattooing my name on his arm, and overwhelming me with sweet texts and calls about how great of a woman I was to him.

I know, I know … *Ria, what in the hell were you thinking moving forward with this guy?* RED flags, sis, everywhere. Well, here's the thing: I was always quick to cut someone else after they wronged me. I gave Kevin another chance because he was the first man I felt loved me for me. He worked hard, I thought he treated me well, and didn't make me feel like I needed to change my appearance. Before Kevin, I never had anyone buy flowers and edible arrangements just because, buy nice random gifts, cook for me, bring me lunch to work, tell me nice things, and appear to be genuine. Damn y'all, that's sad. So I have to ask myself: did I tolerate his bullshit for fear of losing these things … the bare minimum? I guess so.

By September 2021, I was back to work. The gym became a part of my schedule. Working out was my escape from the Kevin nonsense. I was slowly taking time away from the never-ending drama and feeding it elsewhere, my personal transformation and goals. I needed some form of activity in my day-to-day life, so there were no more excuses like before surgery. At work, I would go out for walks during my tour of duty around the clinic. After my commute home, I would walk around the complex or find my second wind to hit the gym for a workout.

The weight loss surgery experience in the beginning was eye-opening. I compared life then and now and couldn't believe the difference. Before, I would quickly give excuses to avoid working on anything for myself. "Oh, I'm too tired. I'd rather get Chipotle and chill." Now, there was a greater sense of commitment to my personal goals: health and career. Not being consumed by food and the desperation to lose weight allowed me to breathe and place more focus on other things like studying for certifications, working without feeling physically miserable, and enjoying runs on the treadmill. I was more energized and ready for anything! This is a plus in my line of work because no days are the same, and you never know what to expect. Before surgery, I was down for lunch runs to Wegmans to grab coffee-flavored shakes or Chick-fil-A spicy chicken sandwiches. Spending hours across the bed to re-watch the *Mindy Project* on Hulu in the midst of a good Bath and Body Works scented candle. Now my life is alkaline water, Premiere shakes, spending time with amazing friends, and plotting my gym missions between working and studying. #balancinghealthy

Reflection:

Like anything we truly desire in life, we have to want it badly enough to commit ourselves to it. Great athletes like Michael Jordan and Serena Williams practiced day in and day out, not just before the big game. It was a part of their everyday routine. Consider studying to graduate, taking additional courses for certifications, or how entrepreneurs pour themselves into their vision around the clock to become successful.

I've committed myself to the process of physical self-improvement that will affect my emotional and mental mood also. It's a never say die, 24-hour relationship you develop with the most important person in your life. YOU. From the first drink of water in the morning to the last vitamin in the evening. After the worst tour of duty, I still found energy to strip those scrubs off, throw on my baggy American Eagle tie-dye sweats, and hit the treadmill. I didn't want to, but I needed to. The endorphin release kept me sane and welcomed my new slender frame, plain and simple.

While welcoming change in my physical life, I was understanding change in relationships is unavoidable. Perhaps it's God's way of saving you. Consider it your Training Day. Remember that gritty, gangster, Denzel Washington movie where he put baby boy, Ethan Hawke, through the ringer? God is ultimately preparing you for what you need versus what or who you think you want. I'd been hibernating for too long, physically and emotionally. Now, I'm ready to welcome everything God is ready to bless me with. New experiences that will hopefully help someone else, new doors to walk through, and memories I will not forget.

When life throws you lemons, damn the lemonade. You grab your sunscreen, a folding chair, and make a pitcher of margaritas to your liking. If you're going through some shit for a while, might as well make the most of it! Seriously, this is what you are going to do *and* at the same time: nothing and something. Nothing negative to seek revenge. God will handle this for you on His own time. As angry as you are or how badly you want someone to feel the pain they have caused you, it is not your assignment to hurt them. I know it seems like it will feel good in the moment, and I will not lie to you, it does—a short-lived moment of vindication (ex: slashing a tire or bleaching clothes). Unfortunately, nothing changes what happened. You will still hurt until you heal. But what you will do is something, whatever will benefit you in the brightest internal light, restore the imbalance of justice, and help you discover peace again.

In life we meet some really amazing people, and then we meet some really horrible ones, but either way they teach us valuable lessons, okay? For the people who have misled you, lied to you (played crazy in your face), mishandled you, made you feel less than, had you thinking you were crazy for a minute, or took your kindness for weakness, appreciate the experience after the shit storm of love passes over. You have learned the biggest lesson about yourself: YOU are naturally that wholesome of a person. It intimidates the weak and exposes the insecurities of others. Truthfully, you two were never on the same level and never will be. Your heart is as pure as gold, and their heart is whatever it needs to be to get what they want in any moment. YOU had to go through a certain level of pain to understand your self-worth and start living up to it, sorry kid. That relationship did not work out for you because God has something (and someone) better planned for you. Settling for less than what your heart deserves will be on you if you stay, so be brave enough to walk away to prepare for what is really yours: respect, honesty, loyalty, and someone who genuinely adores you, good, bad, and indifferent. Baby, trust me, the next person who comes into my life gotta be that good, healthy, and crazy about me. Okay!

Journal Question:

Think about one of the most challenging moments in your life. Who was your support system and why?

_____

_____

_____

_____

_____

_____

_____

_____

_____

_____

_____

_____

_____

_____

_____

_____

_____

_____

_____

_____

_____

_____

"Every woman that finally figured out her worth has
picked up her suitcases of pride and boarded a flight to
freedom, which landed in the valley of change."
—Shannon L. Alder

Chapter 28

The Funeral and The Boxing Ring

Dominique

After my breakup with Cedric, I found myself entertaining good ol' faithful Ishmael. He gave me his usual speech and promised he'd changed and was ready to be a family. I see now that the constant judgment I'd received from Cedric left me vulnerable, and I tricked myself into thinking Ishmael was the only man who would accept me for me.

Man, do I wish I would have bypassed the events that took place next. I was tired of dating and felt guilty for not giving my children the family I felt they deserved. To give our relationship my all, I was willing to overlook all of Ishmael's past offenses. Unfortunately, it only took two to three months for Ishmael to show his true colors and revert to his old ways.

It was Christmas Eve, and I had bought Ishmael multiple Christmas gifts from myself and the kids. He stopped over for a few minutes and promised to come back the next day, so we could spend Christmas together as a family. I noticed he had become distant so I asked him why. He told me he was grieving the recent death of his grandmother. Mindful of his recent loss, I refrained from being selfish and starting an argument over my suspicions.

Christmas Day came and went without as much as a phone call from Ishmael. He was nowhere to be found, per usual. My children and I waited for him to come over. I called repeatedly, with his phone going straight to voicemail. At that moment, I realized Ishmael hadn't changed, and I was reliving painful memories from our past. Triggered, I promised I would never allow myself to feel these emotions again.

Days went by, and still no word from Ishmael. I was left with the disappointment on my children's faces of not seeing their father, yet another promise he didn't keep.

I knew his grandmother's funeral was on December 29, and I questioned if I should attend. I remember talking to my best friend on the phone the morning of, still unsure of my decision. For some reason, I had an unsettling feeling that something was going to happen at this funeral. I told Ria, "What if he shows up to the funeral with another woman?" Then I laughed and said, "Ishmael isn't that stupid!" Little did I know then how important it is to listen to that small still voice that is a forewarning for what is to come. To avoid any conflict, I asked my mother to attend the funeral with me. Despite my feelings for Ishmael, I wanted to pay my respects to his family, who had become family to me over the fifteen-plus years we knew each other.

Now, remember when I told you I have a reputation for coming to blows at funerals? Well, here is one reason why. My mother and I walked into the funeral home. Everything appeared to be fine. I sat in the back, planning my exit. People walked up to me, asking where Ishmael was. I shook my head and told them their guess was as good as mine. No more than ten minutes later, here comes Ishmael walking through the door with Samantha.

I was stunned. Not only was he with another woman, but she was white. Now, I know what you're thinking. I am not racist, nor do I have anything against interracial dating, but to me, this was a slap in the face. Samantha was screaming "trailer park," if you know what I mean. My mind was racing with thoughts of betrayal that I and several other black women had endured due to Ishmael's lies. But here he was with her, smiling like she was his new trophy and he'd hit the lottery.

I felt ready to explode, and suddenly, Ishmael looked at me and whispered, "What's up, Nique?"

All I saw was red! *The audacity of this bastard*, I thought. I looked at my mother and asked her to tap him on the shoulder so we could talk. She looked at me as a fellow Cancerian and said, "You don't need to cause any drama at this funeral!"

I promised her I just wanted to talk. Ishmael and I walked into the hallway, and I asked him if we could go outside to chat. We walked to the corner, and I asked him, "Who is the woman you brought with you?" He looked at me with a smirk on his face and said, "Oh, she's just a friend who wanted to support me." Disgusted, I asked how he could be so disrespectful. He stepped closer and said, "I didn't invite you and didn't know you would be here."

Without thinking, I clenched my fist and attempted to punch him in the face. He ducked and dodged my first punch. But that didn't stop me. I grabbed him by his collar when his cousin Cookie came out of the funeral home running. She grabbed my hand and begged me to stop. At that moment, I felt I was a hunter and would not stop until I devoured my prey. Before I knew it, the entire funeral had moved outside to watch the show. Ashamed, embarrassed, and hysterical, I left the funeral. I felt stupid and betrayed.

Hours later, Ishmael called me, laughing. He promised me he loved me and said I was the one. He tried his best to convince me that I had overreacted. For me, this was the last straw. Ishmael viewed my tears and heartbreak as a game. Due to his lies and failure to control my emotions, I realized I would end up in jail and lose everything I had worked so hard for.

Reflection:

Several days after the funeral, I apologized to Ishmael's family for my actions. They accepted my apology and assured me no love was lost. They had witnessed the woes of our relationship and advised me to get as far away from him as I could. They saw how unhealthy we were for each other. We found comfort in the dysfunction of our relationship. Ishmael had a vengeful mindset. Despite all he put me through with the number of children he had behind my back and constant cheating, my relationship with Cedric left him with a vendetta against me. He explained to me that true love doesn't walk away but accepts and tolerates the pain experienced in an unhealthy and toxic relationship. This is a "*lie*," okay! No woman, man, or person should have to go through hell to prove her worth or loyalty to a man.

Let's flashback, a year prior to this incident and during my relationship with Cedric, Ishmael became enraged. Cedric and I had just left my aunt's 60th birthday bash, and we were sitting on my couch talking and cuddling, when my phone rang at 2:00 am. I jumped up, startled, and answered the phone. Ishmael was on the other end yelling and telling me to come outside. He accused me of being a whore and asked if my kids were at home. Cedric saw the horror on my face and went into protective mode, as Ishmael began to threaten our safety. He walked around the house and banged on my family room windows. Livid, Cedric got up quickly and darted for the door. I ran after him and begged him to stay in the house with me, knowing Ishmael carried a concealed weapon. If Cedric had gone outside, I feared how detrimental the situation could become. Terrified, I thought, *He's going to kill us both.* I was also embarrassed and had never seen Ishmael act so erratically. After calming Cedric down, I begged him to spend the night to ensure his safety. The last thing I wanted was to be held responsible for my ex's heinous actions. Sleepless, I remember calling my cousin to pray with me. I was on edge.

The next morning, I received several blocked calls. When I answered, Ishmael again accused me of being a slut and told me how much he hated me. In complete shock, I was lost for words and hung up the phone. I had given Ishmael everything: my love, virginity, first daughter and son, money, and most of all my peace. And after all he had put me through, he hated me! Wow, I thought it was good for him. Although unintentional, it felt good knowing he got a taste of his own medicine and experienced a small glimpse of what he put me through. Everything was about him. What a narcissist! He used our altercation at the funeral as payback. Once again he longed to humiliate me, and I let him. For so long I gave him the power to control my emotions.

My parents are far from perfect, but I never saw my mother degrade herself or compete with other women for my father's attention. While growing up, my father made sure we knew he only had room for the three women in his life: my mother, my sister, and me. I yearned for that same sense of security and loyalty.

After the funeral, I hid from my family because I had stooped to an all-time low. After days of avoiding calls and a lecture from my parents, my father was in the hospital experiencing chest pain. While in the hospital, my father looked at me and said, "Don't ever chase someone who isn't willing to chase you back." His words resonated with me like never before. I realized the role I played in this cycle of destruction and insanity. I understood that I had to look within and pinpoint why I allowed someone to inflict such disrespect and pain in my life for years. It is true that one can only treat us the way we allow them to.

That day moving forward, I chose to respect myself and demand the same from others. This is one event in my life I would like to go back in time to erase. However, I understand mistakes are a necessary part of life. Mistakes, if interpreted correctly, are the moments of truth that can launch us into our destinies. The lifelong lessons that can alter our perception and change the negative path we are on.

Listen to your gut and trust the small still voice that I believe is God. Heed your warnings and avoid the embarrassing situations I have found myself in. You deserve better! Anyone who doesn't protect your heart is not worthy of your love or attention.

Journal Question:

What was your breaking point in an unhealthy relationship? When did you realize it was time to choose your sanity over love?

_____

_____

_____

_____

_____

_____

_____

_____

_____

_____

_____

_____

_____

_____

_____

_____

_____

_____

_____

_____

_____

_____

"Learn from your mistakes. Take
responsibility and forgive yourself."
—Ariana Grande

Chapter 29

A Real Live "Thriller"

———

Ria

After a weekend in Atlanta at Invest Fest, August 2021, and making amazing connections, weeks went by and conversations between Kevin and I were beyond a gray area, reaching a "working on our relationship engaged" status. You've learned in previous chapters when I love, I love hard ... *All in* until the absolute end. I mean, this was the same man who had loved me from the beginning, never tried to change or sway my appearance. Now has he always complimented me? He did, in the beginning. But after a while, I felt like I was searching for his visual stamp of approval. When I dressed up for events, I was looking for the "Damn, you look good" right after coming out of the bedroom or bathroom. Often, I found myself mentioning this midway through an event, and his response was, "You didn't even give me a chance ..." Oh okay.

During the start of my weight loss post-surgery, he'd made some eye-opening comments, like "Well, you did this for you," or "Yeah, I hope she doesn't lose any more weight," if someone complimented me on my progress. He never offered sincere congratulations or supportive words of encouragement to keep going. Replaying these statements in my head made me think he was feeling some kind of way, and if so, why? In the past, he would say, "Why don't you ever wear lingerie?" I would sit back and think,

Well, I don't even know if I appeal to you with clothes on. Let alone my clothes off with strings and lace. Women typically do not enjoy searching for compliments. We love hearing our significant other dropping those words of affirmations out of the blue!

My post-surgery weight loss had given me a revised self-esteem, trading in my hi-cut brief Victoria Secret panties for different styles like lacey hipsters. One problem I encountered was having no one to wear them for but myself. The most exciting point in my life became the loneliest. Away from family, friends, and the one barely holding a place in my heart, Kevin. I looked at my fellow IG weight-loss rockstars and admired how supportive their mates were. Meanwhile, what's-his-name would barely drop a heartfelt emoji under mine.

"Is this my life right now?" There I was in Virginia Beach, solo living on the upper balcony sipping small shot glass sizes of Stella Rosa wine. But don't feel bad for me, oh hell no. I take full responsibility for my part in this undocumented YouTube series of "What Now, Kevin?" I'm just shedding light on some of the dim hours of my evenings in the state for lovers.

The final events during Kevin's and my last six months were ones I could not wrap my head around for the longest time: deciding to play house with his "business partner" while convincing me he had a condo just for "us" that needed repairs upon my return to Cleveland; sharing locations with me via cell phone while on "business trips" with his "business partner;" stealing the engagement ring from me while I was at work. I mean, "kick me while I'm down" is one thing but refusing to let me up for air is another. Initially, I held myself together pretty damn good until I couldn't. My breaking point reared its own head as I departed Virginia that cold day in February of 2022. Mad as hell, looking at the heavy-ass container of clothing he left behind in the storage unit for me to collect, I politely poured Drano all through it. Yes, the hell I did. I thought, *You dirty ass b***h ... after all the mishandling of me and wasting my time you're lucky this is all I'm doing.* Considering everything you've done, it could've been worse.

What I learned in my own version of "Thriller" is how to make the most of an unsettling situation. My mind is constantly going, waking up before the alarm clock, and fighting the need to rest at night. Through my post op process, I refused to let my bipolar relationship deflate me completely. What really motivated me in the upcoming months were Kevin's words during a conversation we had during his last visit to Virginia Beach in late July 2021: "Ria, we're just not on the same level." (As if he were on a greater level than I). Can you imagine how dumbfounded I was? I promised myself he would be the last person I lay next to at night to EVER tell me that.

Before surgery, I created a new Instagram page dedicated to my bariatric surgery journey, "@Reggievsgbound," and said I would just go with the flow. I started posting videos, pictures, and quotes documenting my story pre- and post "big day" journey. During a chill afternoon in late summer 2021, there was a period of self-reflection about where I've been and where I'm going. All the gyms, trainers, workout classes, and money I've invested into trying to become a better version of myself: a LOT of time, well-intended energy, and money! Gym membership is about $22/month, boot camps $50-$150/ month, personal trainer $100/week, diet pills $10-$100 per bottle.

In the midst of everything going wrong, I focused on what could go right. For the last twenty-plus years, I've been on the alternating path to wellness. Who better to help someone struggling with feeling overweight or being clinically obese? What better person to motivate someone attempting to approach the starting line to a healthier lifestyle? Some people feel intimidated by perfect bodies or are unable to afford extravagant pricing, causing hesitation with personal training. I want people to feel comfortable and confident, presenting an affordable healthy program they can succeed in.

Sooo … I did a "thing" and studied to become a certified personal trainer and nutrition coach (that was a bonus certificate and much needed). I researched online certification programs and signed up for ISSA (International Sports Science Association). Pricing was great with self-paced courses, and it was a step toward my vision of helping others. I am no Olympic Gold trainer, but I absolutely love offering support to people trying to figure it out! That's half the battle.

It is necessary to be transparent in sharing my experiences with other people, products I've incorporated into my daily routine, and information from my nutritionist in pre-op. Anytime we discover what works or not so much, it shouldn't be held under lock and key; share that knowledge so others can win too! If the universe gives to you, it is your responsibility to give back. This is where I find fulfillment.

Reflection:

Buddha once said, "Three things cannot be hidden: the sun, the moon, and the truth." You know the old saying: When people show you who they are the first time, believe them. Well, I didn't do that. The relationship with my ex-fiancé, Kevin, can be compared to visiting a specialty grocery store, expecting to find a couple different items to bake a cake. As soon as you walk the aisles, all you see are shelves full of condiments and spices, but you keep looking, expecting to find ingredients for your cake. We have all done this.

My past relationships left me coldhearted in the end (picture Omarion singing "Icebox."). When the person did something reprehensible in my eyes, that was it. I cut them off. No second chance to give an explanation or reclaim their position with me. When speaking about relationship red flags, Karen Salerno, MSSA, LISW-S says we need to pay attention to people's behavior. Salerno says, "There's going to be a pattern. Typically, there's not going to be an isolated incident. There will be multiple things that come up." (Salerno, 2022). Reflecting on Kevin's and my love story, there were questionable events from the start.

Over the years, we'd had our share of growing pains. I certainly had my fair share of issues that I was open about early in the relationship: Trust was a huge issue for me. After the initial infidelity, I forgave him, but did I let him live it down? No. I would slide in snarky comments at opportune moments and check his phone on occasion. I was super emotional in my responses toward everything, which never got me far with him. There were times I would become so enraged I would throw things (not at Kevin) in moments of pure frustration, feeling unheard when I was literally telling the man how something made me feel. He would sit there unphased, taking me from zero to one hundred. This was poor impulse control on my end. We needed therapy years ago, individually and as a couple. However, despite our "minor" issues early on, he proposed unexpectedly on a beautiful island in Hawaii. The rest would be happily ever after—until it wasn't. Two people just going with the flow, doing one of two things at the same time: not acknowledging issues and just throwing a band-aid on top of a laceration that needed debridement with sutures and a course of antibiotics.

Salerno also provides readers with a guideline of what a healthy relationship contains: mutual respect, communication without the fear of retaliation, honesty, accountability, trust, support, and fair negotiation. These are key ingredients to any important relationship in your life: family, friend, professional, business, and romantic. Without establishing what these words mean for everyone involved, you are going into a partnership blindly. If it's family, the dynamic could always be complex or toxic if one of the key ingredients is missing or weak. Take a moment to consider what these key terms mean to you. We all need to take time and define these for ourselves first before we go around expecting to connect with everyone else.

By the end of summer 2021, I had never felt more embarrassed, ashamed, and just heartbroken, almost not recognizing the reflection in the mirror. It had been clear for months I was fighting for something that did not exist: a healthy reciprocal relationship filled with love, respect, and loyalty/honesty. I paced the living room after many long days of work, smoking my organic American Spirits, wondering if the last six years of my life were even real? Hell, I didn't know this man any more than the guy who sat at the intersection of Indian River Road asking for change every morning in front of the WaWa gas station.

If there comes a time you start asking yourself questions similar to the ones I mention above while in a relationship, consider letting it go. No, it isn't easy, and yes, the people who love you have been telling you for months or years to walk away. It may take you a while to get emotionally or mentally prepared to get here, but the longer you wait the longer you are strapped in for a ride of plot twists that won't make you feel great. Realize there is no end to this roller coaster ride, and the movie will never have a happy ending. Please save yourself by jumping off the hot mess express and into peace. It will be the best fall you take because you are finally saving yourself.

You've tried meeting the person halfway, attempted to fulfill their requests, rearranged your schedule, relaxed your "crazy" responses to situations, and still you get nothing in return? Ohhh, it's time to go. You entered a space allowing this person to cross your boundaries, giving them green lights to treat you however suits their needs at any moment. Yes, it works out great for them, fulfilling whatever they need on a particular day, but where

does it leave you? I will tell you where ... miserable, sad, and f*****g livid!
Listen up and close, sometimes the right package will end up at the wrong
address. Baby, you are the gift and just too damn good to be accepted by
anything less.]

Trust me, the woman or man God wants to receive you is out there
praying the same Ciara or Russell Wilson prayer right now, babe! You two
are waiting on a few things to happen first. Since you are waiting together,
here is what you should be doing:

1. Take time alone to reflect on what has happened and clear your
   spaces (emotional, mental, and physical) of the past with that
   person.
2. Focus on yourself, working on short-term goals and considering
   long-term goals.
3. Spend time with people who care about you (laugh a lot).
4. Forgive and let go (this may be really challenging for some).
5. Work on healing and being happy (you so deserve it).

"And then one day there you were, shining brightly.
Showing me that I wasn't meant to stay in the dark."
—J.M. Storm

Journal Question:

Think back to your last break up, separation, or divorce. How did you handle the event? What would you do differently? What advice would you give to someone going through this right now?

_____

_____

_____

_____

_____

_____

_____

_____

_____

_____

_____

_____

_____

_____

_____

_____

_____

_____

_____

_____

_____

"Anything and everything you have experienced has been purposeful; it has brought you to where you are now."
—Iyanla Vanzant

Chapter 30

Breath of Fresh Air ... Right on Time

Dominique

In September of 2016, after deciding to cut ties with my children's father for good, I received a DM saying, "Hey, I miss my old friend. How are you?" I looked at the message and thought, *It's Anthony, why not?* But I know what you are thinking. One of those "slide in your DM" types. Right, I thought the same thing! I doubted anything real would happen, so I responded. Things moved slowly, and in the spring of 2017, we had our first date.

You see, we knew each other during my first two years of college at the University of Toledo. As he would say, I played him and did not give him a chance. We were young at the time, and he did not fit into my "ideal" image of a mate. We went on one date, but he was not my type. He had braids, and I always liked a clean-cut guy.

Post-college, we ran into each other periodically, but we were both in long-term relationships with the people we had children with. He had a low haircut and a fresh wardrobe—you know, just grown man-ish. I remember thinking, "Oh, this could work!" But we took our time and reintroduced ourselves to each other. I wasn't thrilled with my weight or belt size, but I was content with wearing a medium blouse and size 12 jeans. We began spending time together and charting new waters. I felt seen and accepted by him. His most appealing quality was his interest in his two daughters. He took the time to spend quality time with them, attend parent teacher conferences and be present. I had never experienced this with Ishmael, and I was intrigued! When he looked at me or showed affection in public, I would blush and feel butterflies. I finally understood how important it is to be vulnerable and allow yourself to heal through the power of love.

I learned that real love is not perfect, and allowing yourself to love again after a heartbreak is a difficult decision. Both Anthony and I were hurt and had years of baggage from our past relationships. Be open with your mate. Do not be afraid to show your heart. You have to be naked, figuratively speaking, to begin the healing process. If you find that they are trustworthy and loyal, let them know about your past and that you are attempting to show yourself and need them to be patient with you. Do not rush a relationship. Build a friendship and truly get to know the person. Anthony and I tried our best to walk into our newfound love with a clean slate and fresh perspective. We discussed every issue as they arose in our relationship. I learned that it is best to be upfront in the beginning to avoid future conflict from issues that have festered and led to feelings of resentment. Adding children to the mix complicates the scenario even more. I wanted to make sure the person I gave my heart to was also invested in my children. Children are both impressionable and vulnerable. As single mothers, it is our job to protect our children by who we allow in their company.

You must unlearn everything you think you know about love, romance, and relationships to let your guard down and allow yourself to love again. At the time, I did not realize the gift God was presenting to me. He was giving me a second chance. Another chance to trust and to give myself for the first time to someone and be vulnerable.

We all make mistakes, but the difference is how we choose to move forward and learn from them.

I'm somewhat of a newlywed. Four years of marriage under our belt, and it hasn't been easy, to say the least—a beautiful baby girl of our own and living amongst the remains of 2020 in our blended reality. Maneuvering through COVID-19 and being black in today's America amidst racial injustice. Life often seems unfair.

I was forced to dig deep into my constant desire to change. After the birth of our first child together, I had gone through a dark time in life. Surrounding the sudden death of my sister, Dawnnay, and the inability to lose weight. I was just unhappy.

I was unhappy with everything in my life, including him. I wanted to revisit the behavior of younger Dominique, the little girl who learned to hurt other people to disguise her pain. After the birth of our daughter, my weight began to creep back up the scale. Like my first two pregnancies, I had immediately lost the baby weight after delivery. I thought I was in the clear this time, too, but boy was I wrong! Over the next six months, I gained back every pound and was heavier than during my pregnancy. As the numbers increased on the scale, I didn't know what else to do. So I turned my anger inward. I remember bashing myself one morning about my weight gain, hating my appearance. At that moment, Anthony stopped, looked at me, and said, "You're beautiful to me. When I look at you, I don't see your weight. I'm not disgusted. I see the woman I love! So, stop beating yourself up!"

The ability to love someone when they won't, don't, or can't love themselves is a gift. We all need someone to rally behind us in these moments when we can't see the light beyond the dark clouds. Whether a parent, friend, partner, or coach, we all need an accountability partner. Today I recognize the need to love myself unconditionally and actively stop bashing myself! We were all made in the image and likeness of God, and that was no mistake!

Reflection:

His words and the look in his eyes showed how visible my insecurities were. I thank him for rallying behind me that day. The ability to love someone when they won't, don't, or can't love themselves is a gift. We all need someone to rally behind us in these moments when we can't see the light beyond the dark clouds. Whether a parent, friend, partner, or coach, we all need an accountability partner. Today I recognize the need to love me unconditionally and actively stop bashing myself! We were all made in the image and likeness of God, and that was no mistake!

I think my biggest gift and curse is my will to be independent. Miss, "I can do it all by myself!" Yeah, no! Can you blame me? I took the world on my shoulders as a single mother, and it affected me in every way. Emotionally, mentally, physically, and spiritually I was drowning. Instead of being honest with myself, I allowed my weight to dictate my happiness and the way I felt about myself far too long. Just now in my late thirties, I am beginning to fully understand who I am, and there is so much more to me than numbers on anyone's scale. Today I am fighting for the young internal me to be free and whole. I'm no longer judging myself and am walking into a new realm of pride.

I had to take a step back and assess my life. As a therapist, we spend most of our day assessing others and providing advice, however, we rarely take the time to create balance in our own lives, at least this rings true for me. I realized that I too would benefit from seeking therapy for myself, And I wondered if I was unconsciously sabotaging myself. Was I still dealing with childhood issues of rejection? Did I fear being loved or accepted? As I began to dig deep, I confronted many of the lessons shared with you. I began to ask myself, "Why do you want to lose weight? To be healthy or was my intention solely based on physical appearance?

Today I want to lose weight, not for acceptance or to meet someone else's definition of "attractive," but to feel GOOD. I pay attention to how my clothes fit, how my skin looks. I would rather feel good than look good and feel terrible internally. You know, to be healthy and live long enough to raise my children into superhumans and become their children's grandmother. I have wasted too much time allowing my weight to interfere with me being ME.

I also began to dig deep into my ability to communicate and my feelings of anger that often arise during conflict. Everyday I am working on my inner woman. I no longer want to be reactive but proactive in my emotions. For the majority of my life, I have acted out of some emotion that usually led to negative consequences. Now I value the woman I show my children. I want them to respect me and not question my ability to make sound judgments. I want to be level-headed and patient. Everyday I take time to breathe and invest in myself. Whether that be getting my hair done, a massage, manicure and pedicure, doctor's appointment, shopping, or lunch with friends.

Self-care is crucial to our overall health. I surround myself with people who want to see me win and not talk about me.

Understanding the perfect version of myself is who God created me to be, flawed and all. Imperfectly Me!

Journal Question:

Who is your cheerleader? Who supports you when you feel down? Having a healthy support system is key in our healing journey. Our support system lifts us up but also holds us accountable.

_____

_____

_____

_____

_____

_____

_____

_____

_____

_____

_____

_____

_____

_____

_____

_____

_____

_____

_____

"How amazing it is to find someone who wants to hear
about all the things that go on in your head."
—Nina LaCour

Chapter 31

The Day Everything Changed

Dominique

F ebruary 26, 2020, was the worst day of my life. I woke up to a 5 a.m. phone call with my father on the other end gasping for air. My father is a big, Barry White type who has always been a pillar of strength in our family. I remember holding the phone, afraid for him to finish his sentence. While crying, my father yelled, "God! Dominique, Dawnnay is dead."

I immediately fell to the ground and thought about the argument my sister and I hadn't fully resolved. Now she is gone. Every memory, every thought came racing back like a flood. As a grief counselor, I understood the reality I was now faced with.

Working in the world of grief and loss, I often wondered who or what my first significant loss would be. I never imagined it would be my sister. For the majority of my life, she was my hero. Don't get me wrong. We fought, fell out, and experienced the normal sibling rivalry, but I always knew she had my best interests at heart. She was my first friend and protector. She understood me and shared my story. When she died, I felt lost and the pressure of feeling alone in this world.

As a younger sibling, you never fully know what it is like to be alone. You always have a partner in crime, a playmate, and more. Even with the six-year gap between us, it was just the two of us. We shared a love for writing, sarcasm, and fashion. Flawed and all, we were sisters, and that was taken from me too soon.

Hours after learning about her death, my mother, two aunts, and I jumped on a plane to Henderson, Nevada, to identify her body. We arrived at the morgue to hear they had transferred her body to a local funeral home. Disgusted, tired, and infuriated, I sat up most of the night wondering what was next. The following morning, we arrived at the funeral home. I stood there in shock as the tears rolled down my face. I looked at her swollen body and cried. The coroner's report indicated she died of an asthma attack. I remember holding my mother and wishing it was all a dream. Emotionally, mentally, and spiritually I was crashing. Angry, I questioned why.

"Why my sister? Why my family!" I cried. Weeks after her death, I found myself questioning my own mortality, and I refused to live a life with regret. I promised myself I would live not only for myself but for her.

Days later, I questioned why I was still in a job that I hated and had outgrown. Although I loved working with my students, something was missing. I felt I had wasted three years of my life playing it safe, and for what? I returned to work angry at the world with a pile of work on my desk. Not a sympathy card in sight.

With anger fueling me, COVID-19 hit. The pause I needed. As difficult as the pandemic has been for many, the shutdown saved my life and allowed me to heal. The heartbreak I faced after my sister's death didn't compare to the trivial breakups I experienced in the past.

The world looked different to me. I resented family and friends who didn't show up for my parents and me. Bitter and broken, I had a new perspective on life. I vowed I would no longer put my trust in those who failed to reciprocate the same loyalty or love I gave them. As I drew closer to my immediate family, I realized more than ever who was in my corner. I found that people who were miles away from me in proximity were there for me the most during this time. Especially my Best, Ria G. She called and texted every day. She cried with me and listened to my long, angry venting sessions for months. For that, I will forever be grateful for the authenticity of our friendship and sisterhood.

Through the pain and frustration, I felt motivated. I found that I always rise to the occasion and perform when my back is up against the wall. Therefore, I want to honor my sister's memory and make her proud. I want her to know every prayer, conversation, and argument didn't go unnoticed. I want to make my parents proud and do everything in my power to ease their pain.

Reflection:

A year after her death, I chose to take a leap of faith. I decided to quit my job and bet on myself, using my personal and professional experience to start my private practice specializing in grief and loss.

I have been a therapist for fifteen years and worked in an array of settings, but my seven years as a grief therapist opened my eyes to a skillset and passion I didn't know I possessed. Many would find working in the realm of death and dying to be morbid, but I have found the reward in supporting people during their darkest hour—the very place I found myself two years ago. It was my knowledge and understanding of grief that saved both my parents' lives and mine. My experience taught me the individuality associated with everyone's grief experience. I understood the complexity of grief that most ignore.

When my sister died, so many people ignored my feelings and told me to be strong for my parents. I often thought, "Who will be strong for me?" Their ignorance and words of discouragement replayed in my head for months, not allowing me (a professional who should have known better) to express my true feelings out of a fear of being judged. Yet, I'm thankful their words brought me back to my passion and motivated me to step out of the box and make my dreams a reality.

Today, I have made a choice to choose myself daily and take small leaps of faith to reach my destiny. My life has not gone in the direction I envisioned for myself as a child, but I continue to strive to be better. From the pain of being a single mother to a wife with years of baggage, I am determined to be the best version of myself.

Over the years of having kids, failed crash diets, and workout routines, I have found the importance of loving myself regardless of what version of myself I see in the mirror. Despite my frustration, I am learning the importance of nutrition and more modern medical practices such as functional and naturopathic medicine. I am learning how high dopamine levels are impacting my ability to lose weight and manage stress. When I am stressed, I understand the need to pause instead of eating that donut or little bacon cheeseburger from Five Guys.

Life is too precious to take for granted. I now look at every day as a gift. A gift to raise my children, love, and grow.

Journal Question:

Have you experienced a significant loss in your life? Did that event change the course of your life?

_____

_____

_____

_____

_____

_____

_____

_____

_____

_____

_____

_____

_____

_____

_____

_____

_____

_____

_____

_____

_____

"Death leaves a heartache no one can heal; love
leaves a memory no one can steal."
—Anonymous

_____
_____
_____
_____
_____
_____
_____
_____
_____
_____
_____
_____
_____
_____
_____
_____
_____
_____
_____
_____
_____
_____
_____
_____
_____
_____
_____

Chapter 32

It is What It is

Ria

People will always have something to say, offer an opinion, and make suggestions about your appearance, new job, who you're dating, new home, where you went for your girls trip, etc. Anyone with a social media account can and will, including us at times. When you are ready for change, you will know. It may take an unfavorable encounter with someone, or the day you walk into Old Navy or GAP and you find yourself picking up a bigger size of 30%-off jeans. You may hit a low point where you wake up and no matter how picture-perfect your knotless box braids with impeccable edges look, no matter how many designers are extending the olive branch to the curvier woman or heavier man, you don't feel like you. It's okay. But figure out your new pathway for change.

During life's journey, you will meet people that make you question yourself and what you deserve. The events shared with these bright-eyed, wide-smiling folks can have the propensity to detour, destroy, or serve as the greatest lesson you needed to learn. In the end, you choose the outcome, NOT them. A nice man once said to me, "Don't give people power over your emotions." It's true. While the disappointment, tears, and heartache are very real, give those feelings an expiration date. You are too damn fine, intelligent, and everything amazingly created to be down and out over someone who did not deserve to even know your damn name.

Yes, it will be hard as hell. Yes, it may be unfamiliar to you. There will be unforeseen storms during your transitions: work may be demanding or you're not feeling the gym (ladies, especially on your menstrual cycle feels the absolute worst). It's your off day and it takes everything to drag yourself to workout with a major attitude. You and bae hit a rough patch, tempting you to slide back into old comfort food habits (skip the protein shake and go straight for the Chick-fil-A nuggets, Chick-fil-A sauce on the side). You might slack on your daily water intake; you are bloated and gain five or ten pounds on the scale; look in the mirror and feel defeated if your new Fashionova or Ksubi jeans are still a little tight. But DO NOT quit. Promise us that every day you will look in the mirror, at any size, and love yourself for who you are in the moment. We all fall down in life, but we damn sure have two choices: wallow in the negative self-talk from others, or we get back up swinging harder, more powerful than before. And when you do, stand tall, proud, and give any pessimistic-ass energy the middle finger with a sparkle of a big girl or big boy attitude.

YOU GOT THIS!

Chapter 33

Signing Off

Dominique

For years, our weight has been the annoying friend we can't escape. No matter where I turn, she is there. Weight reminds me of something I can't wear or the limitations I place on myself because I'm overweight. Yet, it amazes me how far we've come in areas of self-acceptance and retail as a culture.

Growing up, we had limited options for plus-size children and women in clothes and shoes. For so long, there was a perception by some that being heavier in size meant sloppy and smelly. No interest in fashion trends or beauty. The only stores that catered to full-figured women were Lane Bryant, The Avenue, and Ashley Stewart, along with your local department stores. Until recently, these stores only carried "plain Jane" or less appealing clothes. Not to mention there were fewer options for an overweight child! Some parents were forced to squeeze their children in adult clothes, ill-fitting their bodies because they were short in stature.

I am proud to live in a time where we have plus-size models and clothing lines opening their closets to women size 12 and up. We no longer look at being plus-size as a social death sentence, feeling gross or unattractive. Instead, we are embracing the idea of beauty in all shapes and sizes. Beauty begins within, magnified by self-confidence.

Sharing our tales in the boxing ring and burning flames with our weight, and the impact it made on our relationships with people has not been easy. It has been an emotional exploration of the past while trying to keep up with our present lives. During our writing process, we've changed addresses, employment, relationship status, and appearance. This has certainly been one hell of a ride. But who you see is who you get. Unapologetically Dominique and Ria, two Cancerian best friends who have accomplished wins, suffered losses, and are ready for whatever comes next. Together we've reflected on life, love, and numbers on the scale. We've loved hard, fell harder. We've put in the work to become these career-oriented women, putting the needs of others before our own and somewhere along the way forgot to nurture ourselves.

Now, we are changing the narrative. Making **us** the priority, focusing on **our** needs, identifying **our** boundaries, and going for what **we** want. The sideline is no longer good enough, we can only take center stage where **we belong** and **so do you**! Our mission is to encourage and provide you with the support and tools that will help you navigate your own healing journey. Whether it be a failed relationship, weight challenges, single parenting, and more. Our goal is to inspire anyone struggling with life and assure you are **not** alone.

As women approaching the age of forty, we realize how the effects of our weight followed us into every friendship and romantic relationship we ever had. We have lived the better part of our lives thus far broken and bruised by teasing and feelings of rejection. We have supported each other and made a conscious decision to fall in love with ourselves and use our voices by sharing triumphs and multiple failures with you. Let us help you avoid some of the pain we endured.

If we made you laugh along the way, well, that is good too! Arnold H. Glasgow, a famous businessman frequently cited in the *Wall Street Journal*, *Forbes*, and the *Chicago Tribune* said, "Laughter is a tranquilizer with no side effects," and we need more of this.

Life is already going to knock us down, so why not smile boldly, and be willing to stand firmly in the midst of the chaos. We appreciate you taking the time to revisit our past, as we uncover previous hurts, while building self-love, confidence and healing. This is **our** truth, and we thank you for traveling with us.

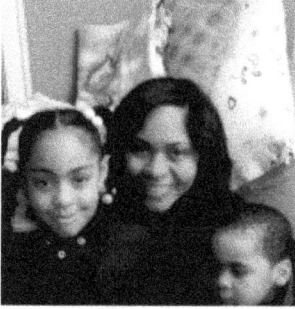
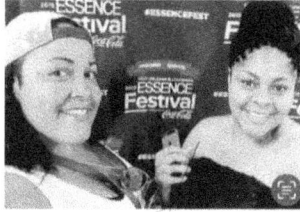
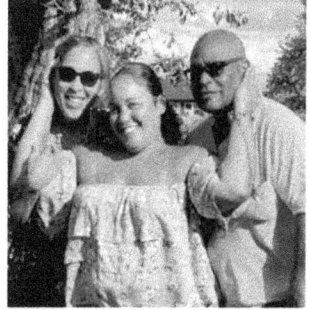
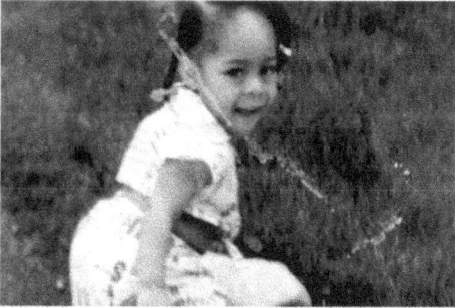
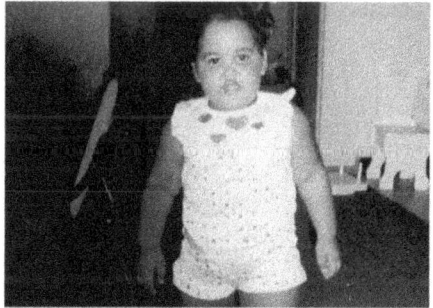
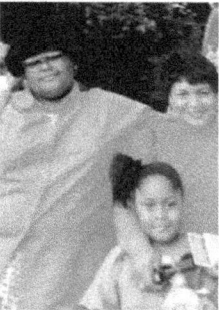
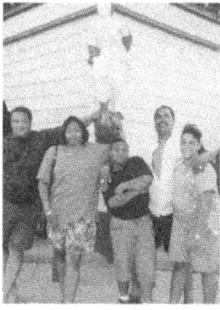
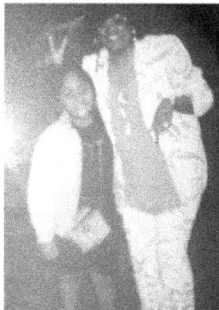
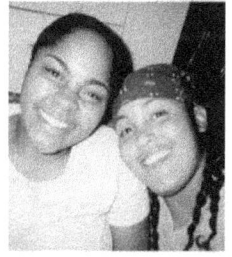

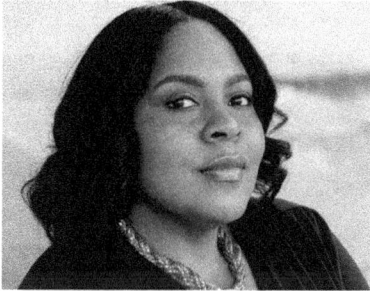

Dominique Toney A testament to her unwavering dedication to helping others and her commitment to personal growth, Dominique Toney's journey begins in Cleveland, Ohio, where her life has been enriched by thriving as a devoted wife, loving mother, cherished daughter, and supportive sister.

From an early age, Dominique exhibited a remarkable ability to offer sage advice and a genuine desire to be of service to others. After completing her education at Regina High School in South Euclid, Ohio, Dominique pursued higher learning at Cleveland State University, earning a Bachelor of Arts degree and continuing her education at Case Western Reserve University, where she obtained a Master's degree in social work. With an impressive sixteen-year career in the mental health and nonprofit sectors, Dominique has established herself as an esteemed clinical therapist, a compassionate grief coach, and an engaging public speaker. Dominique's extensive experience has equipped her with the skills and insights needed to guide others through life's challenges and facilitate personal transformation.

Beyond her professional pursuits, Dominique finds joy in spending quality time with her family and friends, savoring delicious cuisine, and indulging in a bit of retail therapy. Her genuine passion for life, coupled with her resilience, shines through in her partnership with Ria as they embark on a journey of self-discovery, weight loss, and love.

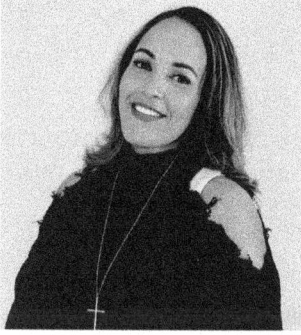

Ria Gibson You will find Ria Gibson in one of two ways: Birkenstocks and scrubs, or skinny jeans and Vans. What you see is who you get. Summer obsessed, taking at least one week off work for peace, tan lines, and mixed drinks, Ria understands that the need to decompress is REAL. When CheapCarribean.com isn't plastered through her phone's search engine weeks before vacay, you'll find Ria just working; sanitizing her cubicle with a Starbucks in hand and a messy bun—ready for whatever.

Birthed in one the greatest Midwest cities; Cleveland, Ohio, Ria hails from the home of go-hard sports fans and the infamous creators of the real Superman, where she grew up on the same street as American comic book writer Jerry Siegel. A proud honors graduate from Regina High school and the University of Cincinnati College of Nursing, Ria is a daughter, sister, auntie, and everything amazing in between. She takes her personal relationships seriously, and her inner circle is tight like her "Seven for All Mankind" jeans. One who works hard, plays hard, and loves harder, Ria's passion for fine dining and true romance turned into a love of McChicken sandwiches and questionable relationships, leading to weight gain and heartbreak. Ria learned some hard life lessons along the way, and found her purpose in helping people save time and energy for the most important person—YOU!

Ria is grateful that her career has enabled her to work in many areas of healthcare, with the one constant being a drive to make a difference, and has embraced new arenas to create change in people. Considered a Cancerian empath, in tune with everyone's emotions more than she can bear at times, Ria has begun her own personal journal on health and wellness, going beyond the physical appearance in the mirror. As she continues her spiritual and mental growth, Ria has found a new and improved self. Her goal is to let people struggling with weight and relationship woes know they are heard, seen, and not alone. Follow Ria on Instagram @reggievsgbound.

References

Beard, Catherine. "How to Keep Commitments to Yourself". *The Blissful Mind*, (2021, March 17). https://theblissfulmind.com/keeping-commitments/

Centers for Disease Control and Prevention. (2021, September 2). *Fast fact: Preventing bullying |violence prevention|injury Center|CDC*. Violence Prevention Youth Violence Bullying Research. https://www.cdc.gov/violenceprevention/youthviolence/bullyingresearch/fastfact.html

Centers for Disease Control and Prevention. (2021, April 2). *Adverse childhood experiences (aces)*. Centers for Disease Control and Prevention. https://www.cdc.gov/violenceprevention/aces/index.html

Lindberg, S. (2022, October 21). *How to stay focused: 10 tips to improve your focus and concentration*. Healthline. https://www.healthline.com/health/mental-health/how-to-stay-focused

Mayo Clinic Staff. (2022, December 13). *Body dysmorphic disorder*. Mayo Clinic. https://www.mayoclinic.org/diseases-conditions/body-dysmorphic-disorder/symptoms-causes/syc-20353938

Salerno, Karen. "How to Spot Relationship Red Flags". Cleveland Clinic Health Essentials (2022, April 7). https://health.clevelandclinic.org/domestic-abuse-how-to-spot-relationship-red-flags/

Sahoo, K., Sahoo, B., Choudhury, A., Sofi, N., Kumar, R., & Bhadoria, A. (2015, April 2). *Childhood obesity: Causes and consequences:*. LWW. https://journals.lww.com/jfmpc/Fulltext/2015/04020/Childhood_obesity__causes_and_consequences.8.aspx

Staff, Familydoctor. org, & Rice, A. (2021, February 26). *Body image issues (children and teens)*. familydoctor.org. https://familydoctor.org/building-your-childs-body-image-and-self-esteem/

Schmidt, J., & Martin, A. (2019). *Appearance teasing and mental health: Gender differences and mediation effects of appearance-based rejection sensitivity and dysmorphic concerns. Frontiers in Psychology, 10,* Article 579. https://doi.org/10.3389/fpsyg.2019.00579

U.S. Department of Health and Human Services. (2023, February 17). *Obesity and African Americans.* Office of Minority Health. https://www.minorityhealth.hhs.gov/omh/browse.aspx?lvl=4&lvlid=25

www.ingramcontent.com/pod-product-compliance
Lightning Source LLC
Chambersburg PA
CBHW022048020426
42335CB00012B/601